ALCOHOL, DRUGS, AND TRAFFIC SAFETY

ALCOHOL, DRUGS, AND TRAFFIC SAFETY

Where Do We Go From Here?

By

FRED B. BENJAMIN, D.M.D., Ph.D.

Formerly, Senior Research Physiologist
Office of Driver and Pedestrian Research
National Highway Traffic Safety Administration
Washington, D.C.

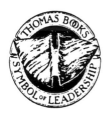

CHARLES C THOMAS • PUBLISHER

Springfield • Illinois • U.S.A.

Published and Distributed Throughout the World by

CHARLES C THOMAS ● PUBLISHER

Bannerstone House

301-327 East Lawrence Avenue, Springfield, Illinois, U.S.A.

© *1980, by* CHARLES C THOMAS ● PUBLISHER

ISBN 0-398-04046-X

Library of Congress Catalog Card Number: 79-28223

Printed in the United States of America
V-R-1

Library of Congress Cataloging in Publication Data

Benjamin, Fred B
    Alcohol, drugs, and traffic safety.

    Bibliography: p. 97
    Includes index.
    1. Drinking and traffic accidents--United States.
2. Drugs and automobile drivers--United States.
3. Traffic safety--United States. I. Title.
HE5620.D7B45   363.1′251   79-28223
ISBN 0-398-04046-X

CONTENTS

Chapter   *Page*

1. INTRODUCTION 3
2. TRAFFIC ACCIDENTS 6
3. DRIVING PERFORMANCE.............................. 24
4. ALCOHOL 34
5. DRUGS AND TRAFFIC SAFETY 44
6. DRUGS AND MEDICAL IMPAIRMENT 71
7. DISCUSSION AND CONCLUSIONS 91

   Bibliography...................................... 97
   Glossary...103
   Index..105

ALCOHOL, DRUGS, AND TRAFFIC SAFETY

Chapter 1

INTRODUCTION

WHEN the Sixth International Conference on Alcohol, Drugs, and Traffic Safety was held in Toronto in 1974, the Addiction Research Foundation issued a special report with the heading: *An International Sense of Frustration*. Things have not changed meantime, and we can look back to some fifteen years of worldwide efforts supported by millions of dollars without significant results.

On the national front, an intensive campaign against alcohol involved accidents was initiated in 1968. During the next ten years, the government spent some 88 million dollars, and the total expenditure (including contributions by the states) was somewhere between 120 and 200 million dollars. Goals were clearly defined in 1968: reduction of the drinking-driving hazard by four-fifths over a period of ten years; 10,000 pedestrian fatalities were to be reduced by 980; 30,000 multiple vehicle fatalities by 9,600; and 25,000 single vehicle fatalities by 9,600, giving a total of 20,180 lives saved every year (65). This was estimated to be equivalent to a saving of 3 billion dollars in accident costs. When introducing this program in his 1969 report to Congress, the Secretary of Transportation mentioned that according to some suggestions, a reduction of the fatality rate of 5 percent per year, leading to a total of 25 percent in 5 years, might be an appropriate measure of success of this program. Obviously, something went wrong. The program did not produce any significant reduction of traffic fatalities (1).

In the area of drugs, the gap between the government program and any effect on traffic safety is even greater.

Drugs other than alcohol were part of the research program of the National Highway Traffic Safety Administration (NHTSA) since 1971. During the past eight years, the government spent over 3 million dollars in the drug-driving area. All the states have some laws prohibiting driving while under the influence of drugs that impair driving performance, but little is being done to enforce these laws. Actually, we do not even know whether therapeutic drugs and drugs of abuse constitute a major traffic safety hazard.* In view of these difficulties, it is not surprising that (except for warning labels) no attempts have been made to develop any drug-driving countermeasures.

On the other hand, we do have evidence that unsafe driving behavior can be changed. In England, the 1968 campaign against the intoxicated driver temporarily lowered fatal accidents by 22 percent and nonfatal accidents by 17 percent. And in this country, the introduction of the 55 mph speed limit lowered fatal accidents by 18 percent. There is also a consistent long-term lowering of fatal accidents. We have a decrease of fatal accidents per 100,000 miles from 7.6 to 3.4 over the last 30 years, but this decrease is due to improvement of cars and of highways, and there is little evidence of any improvement as far as the human element is concerned.

In view of this background information, what is the sense of writing a book about drugs and driving? It does not make much sense to summarize and discuss results that are largely negative. On the one hand, it may be even

---

*Throughout this book, there are occasional criticisms of government policies and activities. This is not intended to blame any person or group. In the government, studies are initiated frequently in response to public or political pressure and not on the basis of adequate knowledge and understanding of the problem. I personally was involved in these programs for many years, and a good number of things discussed in this book were known to us; nothing was being done because there was no provision for this work in the existing plans and programs. In other cases, things became clear to me only when I sat back to write this book.

worse if we try to bypass or even whitewash results we do not like. There is nothing wrong with a negative result as long as we accept it and try to make it a positive contribution to future programs. What is required now is emphasis not on what is known but on what is unknown and how we can get the required information — what was wrong in earlier programs and how can these mistakes be avoided in the future. The book is based on this concept. Failure will not be discussed unless it is in a constructive way, i.e. if there is some way of avoiding this kind of failure in the future. Obviously, it is recognized that this kind of discussion is controversial, and in some cases, the proposed concepts or approaches may be actually disproven by later studies. This is considered acceptable as long as it brings life, hope, and meaning into an area that is now spiritless and full of frustration.

Chapter 2

TRAFFIC ACCIDENTS

BASIC ACCIDENT DATA

THE literature in the drug-driving field is full of contradictions, and frequently such contradictions are due to a different understanding of the problem and different assumptions as to the basic statistical data in the area of alcohol, drugs, and accidents. Tables 1 through 7 will provide the data that will be used as the basis for subsequent discussions. Some of the data are guesswork. When I first considered these problems five years ago, I refused to use guesswork because I thought that we should wait until we had reliable information. As it looks now, we might never have this information for the majority of these problems. The government has detailed five-year research plans, and according to these plans, we will not be much further five years from now than we are at this stage. Therefore, it is considered not only justified but desirable to define conditions that can be used for a systematical approach to the problem, even if the figures may have to be updated if and when information becomes available.

Table 1 presents the total number of accidents for 1978 and the societal costs for these accidents. Many people object to the evaluation of accidents and even human lives in terms of dollars and cents, however, the government needs some way of comparing different types of accidents and the effect of different drugs. Funds are limited, and we need some way of deciding how and where they will be most beneficial. For instance, if drug A increases the incidence of fatal accidents by 2 percent and drug B increases injury accidents by 20 percent, we do need some yardstick for comparative evaluation, and these are the societal costs (43). In this particular case, the societal costs for drug A would be $469,800 and those for drug B would be $112,000. The sequence of total costs is injury accidents, fatal accidents, and property damage accidents.

Table 1

NUMBER AND SOCIETAL COSTS OF ACCIDENTS

| | Accidents | | | |
	Fatal	Injury	Property Damage	Total
Number (**x** 1,000) (44)	48	1,300	15,300	16,600
Costs/Accidents (**$ x** 1,000) (43)	234.9	11.2	0.5	
Total Costs (billions)	11.3	14.56	7.56	33.51
Total Costs (%)	33.7	43.4	22.9	100.

Table 2 presents the corresponding figures for alcohol related accidents. Throughout these discussions, a driver is considered intoxicated if the blood alcohol concentration (BAC) is above 0.1 percent.

In the calculation of alcohol related accidents (Table 3) and those for the drug related accidents, a correction for baseline has been made that needs some explanation. If all intoxicated drivers were sober, they would still have a certain number of accidents. These baseline data have to be deducted from the total incidence of intoxication to derive the damage due to alcohol/drugs. The baseline data were obtained by determining the proportional number from the total number of accidents for the 120 million licensed drivers.

The societal costs for alcohol related accidents are highest for the fatal accidents (Table 4). Next come property damage accidents, but they are distributed over a large

Table 2

NUMBER AND SOCIETAL COSTS OF ALCOHOL RELATED ACCIDENTS

| | Accidents | | | |
	Fatal	Injury	Property Damage	Total
Percent of Total (61)	47	11	5	
Number (**x** 1,000) (44)	21.6	143.	765	930
Costs/Accidents (**x** 1,000) (43)	234.9	11.2	0.5	
Total Costs (billions)	5.1	1.6	3.83	10.53

Table 3

BASELINE FOR ALCOHOL RELATED ACCIDENTS

| | Accidents | | | |
	Fatal	Injury	Property Damage	Total
Mean Incidents of Legal Intoxication in Drivers on the Road*	0.9	0.9	0.9	
Number of Intoxicated Drivers on the Road (**x** 1,000)	0.43	11.7	138	150
Costs/Accidents (**x** 1,000)	234.9	11.2	0.5	
Total Costs (millions)	102	131	68	301

*Assumed.

number of drivers, which would probably limit counter-measures to public education and training.

Tables 5, 6, and 7 give the corresponding data for drug related accidents. In this case, the total costs are lower and the main impact is on injury accidents.

In the evaluation of a potential drug hazard, the correc-

Table 4

CORRECTED NUMBER AND COSTS OF ALCOHOL RELATED ACCIDENTS
(Difference between Table 2 and Table 3)

| | Accidents | | | |
	Fatal	Injury	Property Damage	Total
Number (x 1,000	21.17	131.3	627	779.5
Costs (billions)	5.0	1.47	3.76	10.23

Table 5

NUMBER AND SOCIETAL COSTS OF DRUG RELATED ACCIDENTS

| | Accidents | | | |
	Fatal	Injury	Property Damage	Total
Percent of All Accidents*	15	20	20	
Number (x 1,000)	7.2	260	3,060	3,327
Cost/Accident (x 1,000)	234.9	11.2	0.5	
Total Costs (billions)	1.695	2.912	1.512	6,119

*Assumed values.

tion for baseline (Table 6) becomes much more significant than it is for alcohol. The drug data are obviously controversial, but at the present, we do not have reliable data, and current restrictions on data collection are such that it is not likely that we will be able to obtain this information in the future. The previous figures were developed to provide some hazard assessment for planning purposes, and they are obviously subject to revision.

Table 6

BASELINE FOR DRUG RELATED ACCIDENTS

| | Accidents | | | |
	Fatal	Injury	Property Damage	Total
Percent*	5	5	5	
Number (x 1,000)	2.4	65	765	837
Costs (billions)	0.564	0.728	0.383	1.675

*Assumed values.

Table 7

CORRECTED NUMBER AND COSTS OF DRUG RELATED ACCIDENTS
(Difference Between Table 5 and Table 6)

| | Accidents | | | |
	Fatal	Injury	Damage	Total
Number (x 1,000)	4.8	195	2,295	2,495
Costs (billions)	1.13	2.18	1.13	4.44

One problem that is frequently neglected is the difference between daytime and nighttime in drug use and in accidents. Table 8 shows that there are marked day-night differences between fatal and nonfatal accidents. This is important because the only significant effect of the Alcohol Safety Countermeasures Program was in the area of nighttime accidents (reduction of fatal accidents in twelve of the thirty-five projects). The total incidence of fatal crashes was not affected by this program.

Table 8

THE DAY/NIGHT DISTRIBUTION OF ACCIDENTS
AND OF DRUG USE (PERCENT)

	All Accidents (44)	Fatal Accidents (36)	All Accidents Drugs (44)	Alcohol (36)	Fatal Accidents Drugs (44)	Alcohol (36)
Day: 6 AM to 6 PM	65	46	72	43	64	26
Night: 6 PM to 6 AM	35	54	28	57	46	74

The usage pattern of drugs does not necessarily coincide with that of alcohol. Stimulants are primarily used at night, while sedatives and tranquilizers are largely used during the day. Therefore, it is possible that the effect of stimulants will be primarily on fatal accidents (increase or decrease), while sedatives and tranquilizers are more likely to affect nonfatal accidents (increase or decrease).

THE HAZARD INDEX

There are many factors involved in accident causation, and to be able to develop a cost-effective countermeasure program it is helpful to use a *hazard index* that permits comparative evaluation of various accident parameters.

The following discussion will show that the hazard index used in the past is deficient. Ways of improving the index will be considered.

The controlled method of accident investigation was used by many investigators, including Borkenstein in the Grand Rapids study (9), to determine accident involvement and relative accident responsibility for various blood alcohol concentrations. Subsequently, Perrine (48) and others (19, 20, 32, 35, 50) used the same approach to determine the relative risk of getting involved in a fatal accident. In these studies, the risk is determined by comparing the involvement of alcohol (other drugs, seat belts, etc.) in the accident population with the involvement of alcohol in a control sample collected at the place of the prior accident during the same day of the week and at the same time of the day. The index derived from such a survey is a relative and not an absolute indicator of the hazard involved, and it is an indicator of involvement and not of responsibility for the accidents. These limitations were realized from the beginning.

Soon it became apparent that there was a more basic problem with the index. When the alcohol hazard for nonfatal accidents was compared with the alcohol hazard for fatal accidents, the two turned out to be almost identical except for the very high blood alcohol concentrations. It is difficult to reconcile these observations with the statistical findings that alcohol involvement in nonfatal accidents was about 6 percent compared to about 50 percent in fatal accidents. Further, using the Grand Rapids data it was found that the hazard factor for daytime accidents was about four times greater than the hazard factor for nighttime accidents. In view of these findings, the hazard index was never used to determine the direction and relative distribution of the alcohol countermeasure program. The following represents an attempt to show the cause of the problem with the index and to discuss means of correcting for the deficiency.

The Problem of the Control Sample

Using the traditional approach to a controlled epidemiological accident study, the sampling of the accident population is completely unbiased. However, the sampling of the control is clearly biased. An intentional bias is introduced by trying to limit the sample to the population "at risk." "At risk" for alcohol means nighttime and weekend. For stimulants, daytime may be more important, and for marihuana, the control of age and socioeconomic background may be more important. But the most important bias comes from imposing a characteristic of the accident population on the control. It may be desirable to confine the investigation to at risk drivers, but then the criteria have to be determined beforehand and the same criteria have to be used for the accident as well as for the control population. It may be desirable to restrict the study to rural highways and nighttime. But then any accidents that do not fall within the predefined limits will be neglected, and the control will be selected to represent a cross section of all drivers on rural highways at night.

The accident population can be divided into alcohol involved accidents and non-alcohol accidents.* Similarly, the control population can be divided into sites where the prior accident did involve alcohol (A+ site) and sites where the prior accident did not involve alcohol (A−site). Table 9 shows that the incidence of alcoholism differs considerably between the two sampling sites, especially at the higher blood alcohol concentrations. The difference between the two sampling sites would be of no importance if the distribution of the sites was a characteristic of the sampled population. However, the distribution is being determined by the incidence of alcoholism in the accident population. The result is that with an increase of alcohol use, the incidence of alcoholism in the control increases at a faster rate than in the accident population (Tables 10 and 11). The reason is that the increase of alcoholism in the accident population will be in proportion to the use,

---

*Alcohol is an example. The same would apply to any high risk group, i.e. any blood alcohol concentration, any other drug, any age group, seat belts, etc.

while the control increases in two ways:

1. Increase of the number of alcohol involved sampling sites.
2. Increase of the number of alcohol-positive subjects per sampling site.

Table 9

COMPARATIVE ALCOHOL INVOLVEMENT IN CONTROL SITES
WHERE THE PRIOR ACCIDENT *DID* INVOLVE ALCOHOL
(A + SITE) AND CONTROL SITES WHERE THE PRIOR
ACCIDENT *DID NOT* INVOLVE ALCOHOL (A - SITE)*

		A + Site	A − Site	Total or Mean
BAC 0.1	Number	233	181	414
	Number Positive	13	2	15
	% Positive	5.5	1.1	3.1
BAC 0.05	Number	240	174	414
	Number Positive	34	13	47
	% Positive	14.2	7.4	11.4
BAC 0.01	Number	272	142	414
	Number Positive	88	36	124
	% Positive	32.4	25.4	29.9

*MRI, 1976.

In the Grand Rapids study, the incidence of intoxication decreases as the BAC increases. This means that in the control the number of alcohol involved sites decreases and the risk factor increases. If the same approach is used for the study of drugs, as in a current NHTSA/NIDA supported study, the determination of the risk factor becomes largely a matter of chance. In these studies, if there are 1,000 accidents and the investigator wants to obtain the

Table 10

CONTROLLED ALCOHOL (A) STUDY: LOW ALCOHOL USE (ASSUMED VALUES)

Accident Population	A + Site	A − Site	Total
%	10	90	100
No.	100	900	1,000

Control Population	A + Site	A− Site	Total
%	2.5	0.5	3.0
No.	2.5	4.5	7.0

Old Method: $RF = \dfrac{100 - 7}{7} = 13.3$

New Method: $RF = \dfrac{A \times 10}{C+ \times 1 + C- \times 9} - 1 = \dfrac{100}{2.5 + 4.5} - 1 = 13.3$

same number of controls, he does not go to all accident sites, but he takes a random sample of, say, 100 sites and collects 10 or 20 samples at each site. If the prior accident did not involve drug X, the chances of any drug-positive controls are very low. Therefore, the chances of drug-positive controls depend to a large extent on the off chance of zero, one, or two drug-involved accident sites. Obviously there is a need of making the risk factor more meaningful and better standardized.

The Revised Hazard Index

There are actually two hazard indices, one for the A+ site and one for the A−site. Since the incidence of alcohol-

Table 11

CONTROLLED ALCOHOL (A) STUDY:
HIGH ALCOHOL USE (ASSUMED VALUES)

Accident Population	A + Site	A - Site	Total
%	50	50	100
No.	500	500	1,000
Control Population	A + Site	A- Site	Total
%	12.5	2.5	15.0
No.	62.5	12.5	75.0

Old Method: RF = $\dfrac{500-75}{75}$ = 5.7

New Method: RF = $\dfrac{500}{12.5 + 22.5}$ -1 = 13.3

ism at the A+ site is greater, the hazard index for the A+ site will be lower. Therefore, any increase of alcoholism in the accident population will cause a corresponding lowering of the hazard index. The obvious solution of the problem is the use of a constant ratio of A+ to A− sites that will be applied to all kinds of controlled accident studies.

The question, then, is what should be the ratio? The difference between the two sampling sites is largely due to alcohol, which is a factor that should not be neglected or overemphasized, but it should be controlled. Therefore, a 1:9 ratio (A+:A−) is suggested.

The basic formula is

$$R.F. = \frac{o-e}{e} \text{ or } R.F. = \frac{o}{e} - 1$$

where R.F. = risk factor

o = observed value (accident)

e = control value

The specific formula is as follows:

$$R.F. = \frac{10 \times AA}{1 \times CA+ + 9 \times CA-}$$

where R.F. = risk factor

AA   = percent alcoholism in the accident population

CA+ = percent alcoholism at sites where the prior accident did involve alcohol

CA- = percent alcoholism at sites where the prior accident did *not* involve alcohol

Impact of the Proposed Change

Mainly, the new approach will eliminate the excessive effect of the rate of drug use on the hazard index. However, an increased rate of drug use may have a genuine effect on the hazard index, for instance, by increasing the number of high risk drivers on the road, and this kind of effect will not be eliminated.

The breakdown into sites where the prior accident did or did not involve alcohol or drugs will introduce some additional changes. If the difference between the alcohol/drug involvement at the A+ and A- sites is insignificant, there will be no difference between the old and the new method. If there is a marked difference between the A+ and A- sites and if the incidence of the drug in the accident population is less than 10 percent, the hazard factor will be decreased by the use of the new method. If the differences between the sites is marked and if the incidence of the drug in the accident population is more than 10 percent, then the hazard factor will be increased. Accordingly, it is expected that:

1. The difference of the hazard factor between the fatal and the nonfatal accidents will be markedly increased. This will bring the hazard factor in line with the epidemi-

ological evidence.

2. The difference between the daytime and nighttime hazard factors will be decreased. This will eliminate an experimental finding that had no logical explanation.

3. The hazard factor for the high BAC levels will be decreased, and the factor for the low alcohol levels will be increased. The change emphasizes the safety hazard of the social drinker and de-emphasizes the hazard of the problem drinker.

4. The new method will not require any change for other safety factors (drugs, safety belts, etc.) because there is hardly any information available.

ACCIDENT SURVIVABILITY

The government has a broad and extensive approach to the human element in traffic safety, but there is one area that is not covered and that is low accident survivability (LAS). Accident survival and accident survival rate are important aspects of emergency medical care, but this is postaccident care, which in most cases means prolonged hospitalization, much suffering, and frequently permanent invalidism. What is proposed here is accident survivability as a target for preventive countermeasures.

An accident is fatal if one of the people involved in the accident dies. This may be the driver, a passenger, or a pedestrian. Whether an accident is fatal or not depends on the relationship of extent of injury to accident survivability in the most vulnerable person. If a person with a low accident survivability gets involved in a serious accident, he (she) is likely to succumb where a healthy person would survive. Thus, by his (her) presence, the LAS person converts a nonfatal accident into a fatal accident.

Accident survivability (AS) is the description of a phenomenon that can occur under a great variety of conditions. A significant impairment of any physiological function that is essential for survival will lower the AS. As far as accidents are concerned, three major areas can be identified, and these are (1) advanced age, (2) chronic disease, and (3) alcoholism.

In advanced age, we are likely to find a deterioration of several, or even all, essential physiological functions. A French report (27) comparing people over sixty-five years of age with the general population finds that the average risk of a nonfatal accident was increased by a factor of 1.43 and that of a fatal accident by a factor of 3.18. Another study of the effects of age on accidents (6) shows a steady decline of accident involvement for fatal as well as for nonfatal accidents up to the age of fifty years. Above that age, fatal accidents show a marked increase, while nonfatal accidents continue to decline.

In chronic diseases, one of the essential physiological functions is impaired and provides a point of low resistance. There is no good statistical evidence on the relationship of chronic disease and accident survivability. However, from a medical point of view, AS is equilvalent to surgical risk, and medical as well as surgical textbooks present lengthy discussions on the marked increase of surgical risk in subjects with chronic diseases (49, 69).

Chronic alcoholism is likely to be associated with dehydration, liver disease, and kidney disease which lower the AS. At present, it is questionable whether acute alcohol intoxication (depression of the central nervous system) has a significant effect on the AS. In the intoxicated victim of fatal accidents, a high blood alcohol concentration is mostly associated with chronic alcoholism, and there is no good information available whether acute alcohol intoxication has any harmful effects on accident survival rate. Since alcohol intoxication is similar to surgical anesthesia, we might expect that the surgical risk, which is equivalent to the accident survival rate, is not increased. As far as chronic alcoholism is concerned, Turk (60) reports that more than one-half of the fatally injured drivers as well as the fatally injured pedestrians had liver damage indicative of chronic alcoholism. Filkins (18) examined sixty-seven accidents where one driver was killed and the other driver survived, and where one driver was intoxicated and the other driver sober. You would assume that the intoxicated driver would have a 50 percent chance of survival. Actually it was 12 percent.

Table 12 uses the comparison of alcoholism in fatal accidents with alcoholism in all accidents to show the relative increase of death as the BAC increases. The concept of the LAS will be of value from a traffic safety point of view only if we understand it and can do something about it.

Table 12

COMPARISON OF THE INCIDENCES OF FATAL AND
ALL ACCIDENTS AT VARIOUS BAC LEVELS

Blood Alcohol Concentration gm/100 ml	Fatal Accidents MRI (36)	All Accidents Grand Rapids (9)	Fatal Accidents / All Accidents
0 - .05	47.7	91.0	0.525
.05 - .10	5.4	3.56	1.51
.10 - .15	9.8	2.75	3.56
.15 - .20	11.3	1.76	6.42
.20 - .25	9.1	0.60	15.17
.25 - .30	7.6	0.20	38.0
.30+	9.1	0.12	75.8

A recent survey of alcohol and highway safety (3) indicates a 45 percent involvement of alcohol in fatal accidents, compared with an 11 percent involvement in nonfatal accidents (26). This means that 34 percent of all fatal accidents and 75 percent of all alcohol involved fatal accidents do involve factors that in nature or degree are different from those present in nonfatal accidents.

If we try to determine what could be responsible for the difference between the involvement of these three factors in fatal and nonfatal accidents, we can consider three broad areas:

1. impaired driving performance
2. impaired judgment
3. low accident survivability.

Impaired driving performance may involve perception, night vision, information processing, reflex time, muscular coordination, and fatigability. Nothing that is known indicates that for any of these factors the nature and degree of impairment would be different between fatal and nonfatal accidents.

Impaired judgment involves factors such as overconfidence, decision making, and risk taking. Again, nothing is known as to a difference in the nature and extent of impairment between fatal and nonfatal accidents.

Low accident survivability is by definition limited to fatal accidents. Taking a person of advanced age or an intoxicated chronic drinker, performance as well as judgment will probably be markedly impaired. But there is no evidence indicating that this kind of impairment will have a greater impact on fatal than on nonfatal accidents. However, the LAS will actually take accidents out of the non-fatal category and transfer them into the fatal category.

According to NHTSA estimates, some 15,000 (34 %) of the 46,000 victims of fatal accidents per year are problem drinkers. We would expect them to exhibit some of the signs and symptoms of chronic alcoholism (malnutrition, vitamin B deficiency, acute or chronic pancreatitis, chronic respiratory disturbances, cardiomyopathy, and hematological disturbances). Most of these signs and symptoms are easily recognized. It would be difficult to prove that any of these disturbances are caused by alcohol directly. From a medical or scientific point of view this would be important information, but from a safety point of view the only significant part is the degree and nature of the impaired accident survival rate (ASR), whatever the cause may be.

In the absence of alcohol intake, the alcohol induced low ASR is slowly reversed in younger people, and it is essentially irreversible in older people. For the last eight years the government has tried to attack the alcohol-driving problem by attacking driving performance, and the success was very limited. But would an attack on the low ASR be more promising? There are a number of propitious factors.

1. The low accident survival rate (LASR) is a permanent characteristic of the individual, while intoxication is a temporary status.

2. If "youth" is the target for a countermeasure effort, a person is guilty by belonging to a group. But the LASR driver is a safety hazard on the basis of his own characteristics.

3. In previous programs, the police, judges, and jury tended to be sympathetic to the drinking driver. Intoxication is frequently considered as a temporary lapse that cannot really be condemned; and driving while intoxicated becomes a consequence of the pattern of today's life. The attitude towards the LASR driver is different, and it is expected that the public as well as the police, judges, and juries will be sympathetic to attempts of controlling someone who is a danger to himself and to others. Even the driver can be expected to be more cooperative provided the countermeasures are supportive rather than punitive. Whenever possible, it is probably preferrable to restrict a driver's license rather than to revoke it.

Accident survivability presents a new and important aspect of the drug-driving problem. So far, drugs were evaluated as to impairment of driving performance due to the side effects of the drug, and improvement of driving performance due to the therapeutic effects of the drug. Actually, in chronic conditions such as hypertension and diabetes, therapeutic drugs are likely to improve accident survivability. Therefore, when confronted with a decision whether or not the use of a given drug before driving is indicated, the effect of the drug on accident survivability should be part of the consideration.

Chapter 3

DRIVING PERFORMANCE

THE following is an attempt to present a survey of what is known and what is not known in the field of impaired driving performance.

THE HUMAN ELEMENT IN ACCIDENTS

In 1973, the Institute for Research in Public Safety, Indiana University, conducted a Tri-Level Study of the Causes of Traffic Accidents (58). The study presented a good and systematic analysis of the factors involved in accident causation. Therefore, the following is largely based on the results of this study.

The three levels of the study cover (1) police reports, (2) the report of a team of technicians who were sent to the site of traffic accidents, and (3) a multidisciplinary team that examined 22 percent of the accidents in depth. Table 13 utilizes the third level of investigation only. The figures in Table 13 differ from the original report because the "unknown" was eliminated, and appropriate adjustments were made in the other columns.

As an explanation of the data, it should be pointed out that when going from definite to probable and then to possible, the probability of a single factor will decrease, and the probability of multiple factors will increase.

Looking at the data in Table 13, it is obvious that the human element is by far the most dominant factor in accident causation and may be considered the most promising target for a traffic safety program. However, during the last ten years, a fairly extensive effort, supported by many millions of dollars, was directed toward the impaired driver and did not produce any marked effect on

Table 13

CAUSES OF ACCIDENTS*

	Definite	Probable	Possible
H + E	11.9	28.5	32.7
H + V	1.5	7.9	12.6
V + E	0	0.5	0.5
H + V + E	0.6	3.3	9.8
Human Only (H)	77.8	57.0	44.4
Environment Only (E)	5.7	0.9	0
Vehicle Only (V)	2.5	1.9	0
Any Human Involvement	91.8	96.7	99.5

*Indiana University (24).

traffic accidents, while a similar effort in the vehicle and environment area did produce some significant changes. An analysis of the current status of our knowledge shows some interesting trends that may be important for the planning of countermeasures.

Table 14 indicates that the factors for fatal and nonfatal accidents are similar except for accident survival rate (ASR). By definition, accident survival differentiates fatal from nonfatal accidents. The significance of ASR management as a countermeasure is discussed in Chapter 2. Performance impairment is likely to occur in all conditions and all subjects except in youngsters. Reckless driving, especially speeding, is frequently associated with euphoria, which characteristically is found in youngsters and in acute alcohol intoxication.

NATURE OF PERFORMANCE IMPAIRMENT

The following attempt of identification of the parame-

Table 14

THE HUMAN ELEMENT IN ACCIDENT CAUSATION PARAMETERS
MOST LIKELY TO BE INVOLVED

	Performance Impairment, Including Poor Driving	Reckless Driving, Including Speeding	Low Resistance (Decreased Accident Survival Rate)
Fatal Accidents	X	X	X
Nonfatal Accidents	X	X	
Alcohol Intoxication	X	X	
Chronic Alcoholism	X		X
Medical Impairment	X		X
Drug Effect	X		
Poor Training	X		
Youth		X	

ters of impaired driving performance utilizes some of the information of the 1973 Indiana report (25).

The breakdown of performance follows the physiological stimulus-response pattern. When a stimulus is received by the physiological receptor organ there may be a *perception error.* This occurs when a driver fails to perceive a situation that does require some positive action for the safe completion of the driving task. Such impairment may be due to a temporary impairment of the sensory organ (particle in eye), or it may be due to a permanent disturbance of sensory function (cataract). Perception errors do occur also with improper surveillance. For example, some drugs can produce the phenomenon of tunnel vision.

The next stage is the *recognition error* which occurs when a driver, having received adequate information, fails to see the need for some positive action for the safe completion of the driving task. Examples would be inattention due to sedative drugs or misinterpretation due to psychoactive drugs.

Another aspect of the control of the central nervous system is the decision-making function. *Decision errors* will happen when the driver realizes that some positive driving action is required and selects an improper course of action or takes no action. This is the main point of action for psychoactive drugs and may result in improper directional control, in inadequate speed control, or in improper or inadequate signalling.

The final stage is the motor function. In the case of a *performance error*, the driver knows what action should be taken for the safe completion of the driving task, but due to lack of skill or emotional factors he is unable to take the proper action. Tranquilizers may be responsible for lack or inadequacy of the required action, and stimulants may induce overcompensation.

Therapeutic drugs, by definition, have the task of bringing abnormal function back to normal. Therefore, drug induced impairment is not due to the therapeutic effects of drugs; it is either due to side effects, or it is due to inadequate or excessive drug dosage. This problem will be considered in Chapter 6.

PERFORMANCE TESTING

At present, there is only one legally acceptable evidence of performance impairment and that is the blood alcohol concentration (BAC).

If a performance test (PT) is to be used under a system that recognizes only the BAC tests as legal evidence, the two tests have to be equivalent, which means that the tests are essentially in agreement as to who is legally impaired and who is not impaired. Some tests, such as the Divided Attention Test (39) and Critical Tracking Task (30), assess some major aspect of driving performance, and from a statistical point of view they show a fair relationship to the BAC. However, the intersubject variability of performance at any given BAC level is tremendous. If such a test is set to flunk all drivers at a BAC of 0.1 percent, it is bound to flunk also a certain percentage of the sober driving population; and if the test is set to pass all sober drivers, it will flunk only part of those with a BAC above 0.1 percent (Figure 1). The fault is not necessarily one of the performance testing. The BAC can cause accidents to the extent to that it impairs driving performance.

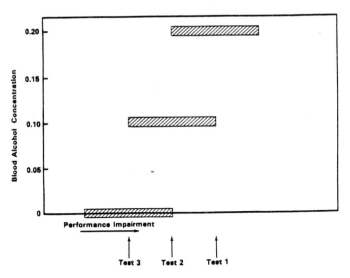

Figure 1: The relationship between tests of driving performance and the blood alcohol concentration (BAC).

If it could be shown that a performance test would be more efficient and also more cost-effective, we could try to change the legal system. The government has conducted a number of studies based on this concept, and the following will present an evaluation of the current status of this effort.

Driving Simulator

A number of driving simulators are currently in operation, some of them highly sophisticated, which makes them expensive in construction, expensive in maintenance, and expensive in operation. However, in these sophisticated devices the user generally reports that the driving experience is very similar to driving on the road. If a visiting congressman has an opportunity to try out such a device, he will surely be convinced that this represents a good investment, but there are marked problems. First, you can run only one subject at a time, and it takes considerable time to obtain a steady level of performance. Therefore, it becomes very time consuming and expensive to run the number of subjects adequate for statistical analysis. In addition, (1) even under optimum conditions the subject is aware that this is a nonhazardous situation; (2) speed is generally controlled in order to standardize test conditions; (3) the factors of alertness, concentration, and attention are different in such an artificial test situation from the routine driving behavior; (4) decision making is difficult to include since none of the currently available methods can be adequately standardized; and (5) the problem (probably the greatest problem with the simulator) of determining the relationship to accident causation presents itself.

Accidents are comparatively rare events. Therefore, investigators have to use some surrogate measure of hazardous driving. But such driving parameters (steering wheel reversal, lane shifting, change of speed, etc.) are poor indicators of the likelihood of accident causation. Moskowitz (40) used a simulator to determine the effect of marihuana on driving performance. Using variation in speed, acceleration, braking, and steering as indicators, he found no effect on car control. He did find some effect of marihuana on perception, which was not part of the driving simulation. Sugarman (59), in a series of 159 tests, determined the effect of alcohol on driving performance. He used lane keeping, speed maintenance, and reaction time as indicators and found a significant correlation between the BAC and performance on each of the simulated driving tasks. This study used the mean of a large number of subjects, and there was no attempt to determine the meaning of differences in performance at any given BAC. Recent simulator studies in Vermont (22) indicate performance impairment at BAC levels between 0.07 percent and 0.10 percent. The latest studies by the same group confirm the findings of a number of accident studies indicating the drivers at high BAC levels (0.08% to 0.15%) have a tendency to drive faster and more recklessly (14). On the whole, simulator studies turned out to be an expensive way to obtain limited information.

In-Traffic Driving Test

An in-traffic driving test is commonly used to evaluate driving performance in licensing but rarely for evaluation of methods that are supposed to impair or improve driving performance. The *instrumented car* is essentially a more sophisticated version of the in-traffic driving test. Again, the test involves a number of problems: (1) conditions are carefully controlled to avoid or decrease the chances of a serious accident; (2) driving behavior is largely determined by the instructor or supervisor, and it is psychologically conditioned by the presence of the supervisor; (3) alertness, concentration, and attention are greatly affected by the test atmosphere instead of the more relaxed atmosphere of routine driving; (4) the driving task cannot be standarized, and comparative evaluation of two or more different conditions requires a large number of tests; (5) decision making is mostly involved but conditions cannot be standardized; and (6) the selection of critical test parameters presents the same problems as it does with the simulator. Parameters such as lane shifting, steering wheel reversal, excessive speed, speed change, and use of brakes have been used as indications of impaired driving performance. Logically, such behavior constitutes hazardous driving, however, at present we have no data indicating the likelihood of such driving behavior actually leading to accidents.

Laboratory Tests

(Field use of these devices is possible but limited by expense and complexity).

Some laboratory tests, such as Divided Attention (39) and Critical Tracking Task (30) do present drivinglike situations, but this means that we have the same problem as found in the driving simulator. We have one fatal accident for every 25 million miles driven, one injury accident for every 1 million miles, and one property damage accident for every 80 thousand miles. Obviously, we cannot afford the time to test for accident causation. Either we have to use unrealistic testing conditions or we have to use some surrogate measures for accident causation. These tests use a combination of the two approaches, and the result is a fairly good relationship to the BAC. However, this does not mean that these tests would be indicative of the performance impairment produced by any other drug. If we want to compare the impairment effect of a number of drugs, we need a test covering all aspects of driving performance that might be involved in accident causation, and the various factors should be weighted according to their significance in accident causation. Such a test should provide objective, quantitative data indicating positive as well as negative changes of driving performance independent of the cause of change.

According to the analysis presented in Chapter 6, a performance test should cover errors of perception, recognition, decision, and performance. But how can we compare a drug that leads to euphoria and speeding to a drug that impairs surveillance? Further, speeding will be more hazardous when combined with poor surveillance, and it will be less of a hazard if it is combined with a fast response time. On the other hand, if poor surveillance is combined with misinterpretation, the combined effect is likely to be less than the sum of the individual factors. First, you have to get the information (surveillance) before you can misinterpret it.

To combine different tests with different units and different variabilities, the tests have to be brought on a common basis. The best way of doing this is by expressing each test in terms of its own standard deviation. The integrated scoring system was used for the evaluation of the impairment of the Gemini astronauts due to prolonged exposure to zero gravity (7). When combining test scores, everything that impairs performance has to be negative, and everything that improves performance has to be positive. For example, in a tracking task, improved performance means fewer errors, but in the development of an integrated score, the sign has to be reversed.

Different parameters of the driving task may vary as to their relative importance in accident causation. For example, decision making is a task that is difficult to measure. The variability is probably marked, and it will be difficult to obtain changes of several standard deviations. On the other hand, response time has a low variability, and a change of several standard deviations might be observed fairly frequently. We could attach a weighting to factors that are important for traffic safety, but this will also increase the effect of chance. If in a given situation decision making comes up with a reading of one standard deviation and if we apply a weighting factor of two, this makes decision making an important contribution to the integrated score, although a reading of one standard deviation may have occurred on the basis of chance only.

This discussion indicates that a meaningful universal test for drug induced performance impairment would be extremely difficult, however, we do know enough about the effects of psychoactive drugs that we can select specific tests for specific drugs. Many literature studies utilize this approach. But most investigators did not realize that this might mean a different test for each drug and that even if the same test was used for two different drugs, the results might not be indicative of the relative difference of driving hazard.

It may be desirable to develop a complete integrated performance test, even if the complete battery of tests would never be used. The availability of a total score makes it easier to select an appropriate system in any specific test situation. Further, such a score would indicate what is the variability of the test compared to the variability of the total driving performance, and it would provide a basis for a crude comparison of different drugs.

Chapter 4

ALCOHOL

ALCOHOL ENFORCEMENT AND
THE PERFORMANCE TEST

IT is now more than fifty years since alcohol has been recognized as a major factor in highway safety. Originally, the evidence of intoxication was based on the behavioral characteristics of the driver, but for the last forty years tests of the blood alcohol concentration (BAC) have gained in prominence, and they are used more and more as court evidence of intoxication. To some extent the shift to the BAC test is illogical. If the alcohol causes accidents, it is only via performance impairment. If there is any divergence between the two parameters, the performance evaluation is bound to show a better correlation to accidents. However, performance, and especially driving related performance, is difficult to evaluate, while the measurement of the blood and breath alcohol concentration is fairly simple; it produces numerical data, and there is a good statistical relationship of the BAC to accidents, especially to fatal accidents.

The BAC test is based on the assumption that at the legal limit of 0.1 percent BAC (0.1 grams of alcohol per 100 ml of blood) *all* drivers are impaired The concept is not unreasonable, though the degree of impairment at 0.1 percent BAC varies. Most drivers are markedly impaired at a much lower BAC. To reach the legal limit you have to consume 4 to 5 twelve ounce bottles of beer or 4 to 5 one and one-half ounce drinks of scotch, brandy, or vodka within one hour before driving. The test is designed so that from a performance point of view the number of false positive tests are minimal, but there are a large number of false negatives, i.e. people who are functionally impaired but legally permitted to drive. The legal limits were designed for enforcement purposes and for that they work very well, but if the concept of legal limits is used in education and training, it is likely to create a hazard. If someone is impaired after two or three drinks, you do not want to tell him: "Legally you are not impaired, and you can even continue and take a few more drinks." The law recognizes that many people are impaired at a BAC between 0.05 percent and 0.1 percent BAC. But practically, you cannot get convicted of driving while intoxicated (DWI) unless you have a BAC of 0.1 percent or higher. As far as enforcement is concerned, consideration may be given to lowering the legal limit. Except for this problem, the system works and there is no reason for change. As far as education and training are concerned, there is a need for basic change.

We allow people to drink before driving, but we do not tell them how much they can safely drink. It is really not surprising that the educational and training approach to alcohol and driving presents a series of failures. The concept of legal limits should be replaced by individual performance limits. If a driver is involved in an accident or if a driver has been speeding and the police officers suspects alcohol intoxication, he wants to confirm his suspicion by a performance test. The usual tests, such as walking a line or picking up a coin are extremely crude. They are suitable only for the detection of advanced impairment; they are not specific for alcohol and are affected by other drugs, by medical impairment, by advanced age, and by fatigue as well. In addition, for an inexperienced drinker these tests are likely to be positive even if the BAC is far below the legal limits, and for a chronic drinker these tests are likely to be negative even if the BAC is significantly above the legal limits.

During the last few years, the NHTSA had several contracts to determine the possible use of the Nystagmus test as an indication of alcohol induced performance impairment. Nystagmus refers to a flicklike movement of the eyes that occurs when the gaze is shifted from one point of interest in the environment to another. When vigilence is suppressed by alcohol, tranquilizers, or fatigue, the velocity and accuracy of eye movement decreases and the reaction time increases. In the 1979 five-year program plan, Nystagmus is described as an accurate indicator of alcohol impairment that may be suitable for roadside testing. It is correct that the test shows a good correlation to the blood alcohol concentration, but it works only if each subject serves as his (her) own control, and each test takes one and one-half to two hours. The NHSTA contractor maintains that the test works also as a fast test in the hands of a police officer, but the actual data show that the tests can only differentiate between sober and legally intoxicated, and finer differences are lost.

What is the solution to the problem? First, the police officer is not interested in impairment but in alcohol intoxication. The legal basis for arrest is the BAC, and that should also be the basis for his test. If it is too expensive to supply an electronic BAC tester to every police officer in the field, it should be possible to use a disposable breath alcohol tester. The test is crude, but it forms a much better basis for an arrest decision than any of the performance tests.

Unfortunately, this kind of test was discredited in 1971 by a publication by R. Prouty and B. O'Neill (51). The investigators showed that these tests have a wide variability, but instead of talking about variability or confidence limits, they talked about false positives and false negatives. In the eyes of the legal community, this completely discredited the test. Scientifically, this is not justified. If a test has 95 percent confidence limit of ± 50 percent, the police officer who makes an arrest only if the BAC reading is above 0.15 percent BAC has a 95 percent chance of being correct, which is much better than anything that can be achieved by the crude performance tests. The NHTSA is working on the improvement of the disposable breath testers, and it is expected that devices that are better than ± 30 percent will soon be available, costing less than five dollars.

A similar problem exists with the Alcohol Safety Interlock System, which is now the Drunk Driver Warning System. In this case, a driver has to perform a skilled task before he can start his car, and the task is supposed to differentiate between intoxicated and sober. The concept is ingenious, and over the last seven years the government has spent millions of dollars for this project, though several people pointed out that there is no legally acceptable solution of the problem. If you set the sensitivity of the device so that it is in compliance with the concept of legal limits (0.1 percent BAC) and flunks all drivers who are legally intoxicated (see Fig.1, Test 3), the test will also flunk many people who are not legally intoxicated and some who are completely sober. If the test is set to pass all sober drivers (see Fig. 1, Test 1), it will also pass many who are legally intoxicated, though the test will flunk all drivers at some higher BAC level.

If the test was used only for chronic drinkers who do not stop drinking until their BAC is above the 0.20 percent BAC level, the test would be effective for this group, but then the test would invalidate the concept that at the 0.1 percent BAC level every driver is intoxicated. No doubt, soon a clever lawyer would show that his client even when legally intoxicated could pass a government test for impaired driving performance. Obviously, if the law defines intoxication in terms of blood or breath alcohol concentration, it would be difficult to do any test for impairment that is not functionally correlated to the blood/breath alcohol concentration. Even if the technical problem could be solved there is the legal problem that may make it impossible to ever use the device. Legally, it would be preferrable to have a device based on the measurement of the breath alcohol concentration, although this approach presents problems of calibration, maintenance, and tamper proving.

EDUCATION AND TRAINING

There was a time when the government had an official policy, "Do not mix drinking and driving." Soon it became apparent that a large section of the driver population did not consider this as acceptable. At the same time we obtained statistical data indicating that limited alcohol intake (below 0.05 percent BAC) does not cause a significant increase of the traffic safety hazard. The official government policy now is that *some* people are *impaired* at a BAC of 0.05 percent, and *all* people are *intoxicated* at a BAC of 0.1 percent. Obviously, the driver wants to know, "Where do *I* fit in?" and there is no answer. The BAC information and the emphasis on legal limits is like selling a car that can reach a speed of 100 mph in a country where the speed limit is 55 mph.

The Alcohol Safety Action Program included a public information campaign that at the peak had a contribution of 32 million dollars worth of advertising. The results showed more awareness of the drinking-driving problem, more knowledge about the blood alcohol concentration and about legal limits, and no significant change in the pattern of alcohol involved traffic accidents. The NHTSA plans for 1980 through 1984 call for $375,000 for public information in the alcohol field and one million dollars for the development of educational material for the states, but the policy and approaches are essentially the same as those used in earlier programs.

A specific example of this approach is the Self-Tester Project. Self-Testers were developed by the government and by some private firms. These devices are set up at a drinking place or on the occasion of a drinking party and allow a driver to test his BAC before driving home. Some of these devices have a numerical display of the BAC reading. This is the most dangerous type because it can lead to competitive drinking. Somewhat better are devices with a color display: red for intoxicated, yellow for impaired, and green for unimpaired. The approach is the same as the one used previously in mass education with no or sometimes negative effects. So it is not surprising that the contractor concluded that the presentation of intoxication levels and related information, as implemented in this study, does not desirably affect drinking-driving behavior. Nonetheless, a new contract was initiated, assuming that a better approach to the subjects might produce more positive results.

The problem in alcohol education and training is not how to disseminate information but what is the information that should be disseminated. Past experience shows that knowing more about the BAC and the legal limits has apparently very little influence on the drinking-driving behavior. The information that is considered most meaningful is the personal safe driving limit. In the past, we had several campaigns based on the slogan, "Know Your Own Limits," but the information provided was based on the BAC and not on performance. It surely did not present a personal safe driving limit, and that is probably why the liquor industry strongly endorsed these limits. To no one's surprise, knowing the BAC limits has no significant effect on the alcohol consumption. The individual performance limits are lower and may well lead to opposition from those who have commercial interest in alcohol consumption. Therefore, some people in the government may be reluctant to adopt such a policy.

If we want to go ahead, the question is how can we provide to the individual driver information as to his state of performance impairment? If we want to come from BAC to impairment, we have to make appropriate corrections for those factors that account for the variability of performance at any given BAC level. The main cause of performance variability is drinking experience. Hurst (23) showed how for the drinking driver the probability of accident involvement decreases with increased drinking experience (Fig. 2). This may be unfortunate because for some people it may be an inducement to drink more or more regularly. But if we want to educate the public as to their safe driving limits, we cannot conceal some facts that are clearly relevant but might induce some people to increase their alcohol consumption.

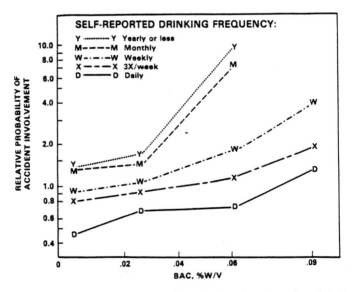

Figure 2: Relative probability of crash involvement (by drinking frequency subgroups) as a function of BAC where 1.0 = relative probability of composite group at zero alcohol. (Hurst, P., 1974)

The following will indicate the principle of the proposed approach. Calculating the legal limits of intoxication, a 170 pound man could consume five one and one-half ounce drinks of whiskey within one hour before driving. To reach the safe driving limits, the following corrections (using assumed figures) would have to be made — for a person who drinks two drinks per year we would deduct three drinks from the legal limit; for two drinks per month we deduct two drinks; for two drinks per week we deduct one and one-half drinks; for two drinks per day we deduct one drink; and for people who drink more than two drinks per day, we accept the legal limits. Further, if the driver is under the influence of sedative drugs or markedly fatigued, any alcohol intake would constitute a safety hazard. If the person had a substantial meal within one hour before driving, he can add one drink to the score, and if drinking started more than one hour before driving he can add one ounce of whiskey for every additional hour.

The communistic countries have a legal limit of 0.02 BAC, which is the concentration where the most sensitive person is supposed to be impaired. From a safety point of view this sounds good, but we do not know how far this policy is actually enforced. In this country we have many more drivers, and it would be extremely difficult to get such a bill passed by Congress, and if passed, to enforce such a policy.

It is always difficult to change human behavior, but it is assumed that a public information campaign that is based on the concept of individual performance impairment will have a much better chance of success than a campaign that stresses the legal limits. The effectiveness of such a campaign may be increased by prohibiting advertising, by increasing taxation, by decreasing the alcohol concentration of commercial products, by developing means of increasing the breakdown in the gastrointestinal tract, and by demonstrating the cancerogenic effects of alcohol. We do have low-caffeine coffee and low-nicotine cigarettes, why not low-alcohol alcohol?

COUNTERMEASURES

The problem with the design of countermeasures is that all the emphasis is on the degree of impairment of the target group, and neglected is the degree of impairment after successful application of the countermeasure. If a driver goes to a drinking party and he comes back in a state of legal intoxication, he is obviously a safety risk with a risk factor of about 20. But the degree of estimated risk and the benefit to be derived from a countermeasure depends on the difference of the degree of impairment before and after application of the countermeasure.

1. If the driver limits his alcohol intake just sufficiently to stay below the legal limits, he will still be markedly impaired (the difference between the supralegal and sublegal levels will be small), and the risk factor may be lowered from 20 to 10.

2. The driver may go to the party but refrain from any alcohol intake; the impairment will be greatly decreased. But a heavy drinker is a safety hazard even when sober. There will still be an increased risk, and the decrease may be from 20 to 4.

3. The risk factor will be decreased slightly more if another person drives who is not a habitual drinker and who did not take any alcohol during the party. The risk factor may decrease from 20 to 2.

4. The reduction of the safety risk would be greatest if the driver cancels the whole trip. In this case, there would not be even the normal risk of driving, and the risk factor would be reduced to zero.

In epidemiological studies, the intoxicated driver is compared with the average driver on the road. This is roughly equivalent to section (1) in the previous example, giving a saving by a factor of 20/2 = 10. However, the campaign of public education is based on the slogan, "Know Your Limits," and the limits are 0.1 percent BAC. Actually, the information supplied to the driver includes the impairment limit of 0.05 percent BAC. But practically, drivers who do decide to limit their alcohol intake do it on the basis of the legal limits and not the impairment limits. Therefore, the benefits of the alcohol countermeasure campaign are almost completely in section (1) of the example with a decreased risk of 2. The result is that there may be a significant decrease of legally intoxicated drivers on the road, but it is unlikely that there will be a significant decrease of total accidents or alcohol involved accidents. When planning a campaign, when projecting the effectiveness of a campaign, and in public propaganda, the effectiveness of a countermeasure is based on the comparison of the legally intoxicated driver with the average driver on the road, resulting in a reduction of the safety risk by a factor of 10, while the actual countermeasure reduced the risk factor by a factor of 2. This happened when planning the 1968 campaign and the same thing happens today.

Chapter 5

DRUGS AND TRAFFIC SAFETY

ALCOHOL AND DRUGS

THE government's approach to the drug problem was largely determined by the approach used for alcohol. Millions were spent trying to develop a drug risk factor and to determine the levels of impairment. Now, eight years after this program was initiated, we cannot show any progress, and there is no chance of doing better in the future if we continue along the same lines. We have to consider the following basic differences between alcohol and other drugs:

1. Alcohol is being taken by people whose driving performance is normal until the alcohol causes the impairment. Therapeutic drugs are taken by people who have some medical disturbance that may affect driving performance. The therapeutic drugs will partially or completely correct the signs and symptoms, which is likely to have a beneficial effect on the accident survival rate and driving performance. However, there may be side effects with harmful effects on driving performance.

2. With alcohol, performance impairment is generally associated with euphoria, resulting in speeding and reckless driving. With other drugs, the driver is mostly conscious of the impairment, and he (she) tends to drive slower and more carefully. Therefore, laboratory evidence of performance impairment may not be indicative of a safety hazard.

3. For alcohol, the only effect on performance is a negative one, and there is a good correlation between the blood alcohol concentration, the degree of impairment as dem-

onstrated in the laboratory, and the likelihood of accident involvement. Therefore, it has been possible to establish legal limits, i.e. a level where every driver is assumed to be too intoxicated for safe driving performance. For therapeutic drugs, the same doses that cause marked performance impairment in an acute user may be a requirement for safe driving in a chronic user.

4. As far as traffic safety is concerned, alcohol is such a dominant factor that it has been possible to develop a complete enforcement program based on blood alcohol concentration only. For therapeutic drugs, multidrug use, and the synergistic or antagonistic efforts, alcohol and fatigue cannot be neglected.

Considering all the points discussed here, it appears to be extremely unlikely that a drug enforcement program similar to the alcohol program can ever be developed. It is considered a waste of government funds if we continue with a program that is aimed toward drug enforcement, although there does not seem to be even a vague chance that this target can ever be achieved.

Extent of Drug Use

In 1967, the California State Highway Patrol (11) analyzed 772 victims of fatal, single vehicle accidents for 6 drugs and found that 13 percent had drugs that could be identified, and another 23 percent had drugs that could be detected but not identified. Mannheimer, in 1968 (34), found that 50 percent of the California population had used some psychoactive drug at least once, and 29 percent had used it during the last 12 months. The study showed that 12 percent of the men and 22 percent of the women reported frequent use. Parry (47) confirmed that 50 percent used drugs at some time. The National Commission on Marihuana and Drug Abuse reported in 1973 (41) that 56 percent of drug involved accidents and 75 percent of all alcohol involved fatal accidents do involve factors that in nature or degree are different from those present in non-fatal accidents. Waller (66) in his analysis of the relationship of medical impairment to driving comes to the conclusion that 15 percent of all drivers have a potential medical handicap, and 15 to 20 percent of all serious crashes are attributable, at least in part, to medical conditions other than alcohol. Haddon also found that natural causes account for the death of 15 to 20 percent of drivers who were at fault in the collision in which they died (19).

Some statistical information on drugs and driving is presented in Tables 15, 16, and 17. This information is based on the records of 1,463,000 drivers and 640 interviews. Of the total population using drugs during the past year, 11.5 percent used illicit drugs, and out of those driving after drug use, 11.6 percent used illicit drugs. Of those who combined drugs with alcohol, 50 percent used illicit drugs, and of those who drove after the combined use of drugs and alcohol, 38 percent used illicit drugs. In view of the synergistic effect of nearly all illicit drugs with alcohol, this may be an indication of a high risk group.

Table 16 indicates that of the marihuana users, 22.3 percent drove after drug use which is 59 percent of the total of those who drove after drug use. But for illicit drug users, the figures are misleading. The combined use of illicit drugs comes to 10.1 percent, which is 26 percent of the total drug users. However, the illicit drug (cocaine, heroin, hallucinogens) users may be half a million compared to some 15 million marihuana users as well as users of tranquilizers.

Table 17 does not provide data for a control group, but the over-the-counter (OTC) group is essentially equivalent to a control group indicating that illicit drugs are apparently not a very significant traffic safety problem.

The Midwest Research Institute (MRI), under contract with the National Highway Traffic Safety Administration,

Table 15

DRUG USE AND DRIVING (PERCENT) (41)

	Used in Past Year	Driving After Use in Past Year
Alcohol	71.9	52.3
OTC* Drugs	68.2	57.6
OTC + Alcohol	9.0	5.9
Prescription Drug	46.3	27.8
Prescription + Alcohol	8.6	6.4
Illicit Drugs	24.2	18.0
Illicit + Alcohol	17.8	13.1

*Over the counter.

Table 16

PERCENT DRIVING AFTER DRUG USE (57)

	Drove in Past Year	Drove Weekly	Drove Daily
Marihuana	22.3	6.6	4.7
Tranquilizers	5.3	0.6	—
Sedatives	4.3	0.8	—
Amphetamines	6.1	1.2	—
Cocaine	2.5	0.2	—
Heroin	2.5	0.2	—
Hallucinogens	5.1	1.0	—

conducted three large studies comparing the incidence of drugs in fatally injured drivers and in drivers on the road (36,37,38). A listing of the drugs found in fatally injured

Table 17

ACCIDENTS AND VIOLATIONS AFTER DRUG USE (PERCENT) (57)

	At Least 1 Ticket/ 3 Years	At Least 1 Accident/ 3 Years
OTC* Drugs	49	53
Prescription Drugs	52	56
Illicit Drugs	65	52

*Over the counter.

drivers is presented in Table 18. The percentages are too low to develop a risk factor for the individual drugs. The risk factor for drug groups is presented in Tables 19 and 20. The variability between the two investigations is so marked that it would be difficult to attach much significance to these findings. The two studies are in fair agreement as to the total drug incidence in fatally injured drivers. However, even with these figures we have to be careful. Some drugs, including marihuana, were not included in the study, and the methods used could discover other drugs such as amphetamine and diazepam only in high concentrations. The data include urinary analysis, and this raises doubts whether the subjects were actually under the influence of the drug at the time of the accident. The 1977 study reports on the incidence of drugs in the blood (Table 21). In the fatally injured drivers, the incidence was 6.06 percent; in the control it was 1.71 with a risk factor of 3.537. In addition to the usual sampling problems there is the possibility of a delay in the collection of the blood samples. For some drugs the concentration may have fallen below the detection limit. In the

Table 18

INCIDENCE OF DRUGS IN FATALLY INJURED DRIVERS
(BLOOD IN ANY CONCENTRATION,
URINE ABOVE 1 MICROGRAM/ML) (36)

Drug	Trade Name	Percent in Fatally Injured Drivers
Amobarbital	Amytal	1.79
Butabarbital	Butisol	0.60
Butobarbital	Butethal	0.60
Diphenylhydrantoin	Dilantin	0.40
Glutethimide	Doriden	0.80
Methaqualone	Quaalude	0.60
Pentobarbital	Nembutal	1.89
Phenobarbital	———	3.98
Secobarbital	Seconal	0.99
Amphetamine	Dexedrine	1.99
Imipramine	Tofranil	0.80
Methamphetamine	Desoxin	2.39
Methylphenidate	Ritalin	0.20
Chlorpheniramine	Chlortrimetone	0.40
Dephenhydramine	Benadryl	0.20
Phenylpropanolamine	Propadrine	2.58
Tripelennamine	Pyribenzamine	0.20
Chlordiazepoxide	Librium	0.80
Chlorpromazine	Thorazine	0.60
Diazepam	Valium	0.60
Meprobamate	Miltown	0.99
Trifluoperazine	Stelazine	0.40
Codeine	———	0.20
Meperidin	Demerol	0.20
Methadone	———	0.40
Morphine	———	0.60
Dimethyltryptamine	DMT	0.40
Lobeline	———	0.60
Quinine	———	0.60

control sample, we have to rely on the voluntary cooperation of the subjects. At best, we might be able to get 85
percent cooperation. But we cannot assume that the 15
percent who refuse cooperation have the same incidence of
drugs as those who donate their blood.

Table 19

COMPARATIVE DATA FOR DRIVERS EVIDENCING
DRUGS AT ANY LEVEL (37)

Drug Type	Living Drivers		Fatally Injured Drivers		Relative Chance of Being Fatally Injured
	No.	Percent	No.	Percent	
Sedatives and Hypnotics	19	2.49	56	11.13	4.47
Stimulants and Antidepressants	1	0.13	27	5.37	40.99
Antihistamines and Decongestants	2	0.26	17	3.38	12.90
Tranquilizers	10	1.31	17	3.38	2.58
Narcotic Analgesics	2	0.26	7	1.39	5.31
Miscellaneous	0	0.00	8	1.59	———
One or More Drugs	32	4.19	89	17.69	4.22
Sample Size	763		503		

The government is just launching another major drug
study. It can be expected that some of the problems of the
earlier studies will be resolved. The methods of analysis
are markedly improved. Reliable quantitative tests for
marihuana are available. The normal clinical blood drug
concentration is now known for all drugs of interest, and
the analysis can be based on the blood drug concentration
of each drug instead of an arbitrary limit of 1 mc/ml. The
control sample can be standardized and additional medical
data can be obtained as required. The main problem that

Table 20

COMPARATIVE DATA FOR ALL DRIVERS EVIDENCING
DRUGS AND FOR WHOM BOTH BLOOD AND
URINE SAMPLES WERE AVAILABLE (38)

Drug Type	Living Drivers No.	Living Drivers Percent	Fatally Injured Drivers No.	Fatally Injured Drivers Percent	Relative Chance of Being Fatally Injured
Sedatives and Hypnotics	20	2.68	30	5.11	1.904
Tranquilizers	3	0.40	4	0.68	1.692
Stimulants and Antidepressants	4	0.54	7	1.19	2.221
Antihistamines and Decongestants	31	4.16	31	5.28	1.269
Narcotic Analgesics	1	0.13	15	2.56	19.042
Hallucinogens	0	0.0	0	0.0	a/
Miscellaneous	3	0.40	6	1.02	2.538
One or More Drugs	59	7.92	84	14.31	1.807
Nicotine	417	55.97	380	64.74	1.210
Salicylates	143	19.19	102	17.38	0.906
Sample Size	745		587		

a/ = indeterminable from the data collected.

cannot be solved is the voluntary participation of control subjects. If it should be possible to use saliva or breath samples instead of blood, the chance of meaningful information would be greatly increased, but if we have a drug concentration of 1 to 2 percent for a given drug group and we have a refusal rate of 10 to 15 percent, the data are meaningless.

The new study is the fourth major government supported drug study. None of the earlier studies were used for any kind of countermeasure development. Even if the information to be derived from the new study was much

Alcohol, Drugs, and Traffic Safety

Table 21

COMPARATIVE DATA FOR ALL DRIVERS EVIDENCING
DRUGS AND FOR WHOM BLOOD
SAMPLES WERE AVAILABLE (38)

Drug Type	Living Drivers No.	Percent	Fatally Injured Drivers No.	Percent	Relative Chance of Being Fatally Injured
Sedatives and Hypnotics	13	1.59	37	4.48	2.819
Tranquilizers	0	0.00	4	0.48	∞
Stimulants and Depressants	0	0.00	2	0.24	∞
Antihistamines and Decongestants	0	0.00	2	0.24	∞
Narcotic Analgesics	0	0.00	4	0.48	∞
Hallucinogens	0	0.00	0	0.00	a/
Miscellaneous	1	0.12	1	0.12	0.990
One or More Drugs	14	1.71	50	6.06	3.537
Nicotine	2	0.24	113	13.70	55.952
Salicylates	87	10.65	78	9.45	0.888
Sample Size	817		825		

a/ = indeterminable from the data collected.

more reliable, it would be difficult to utilize the information for traffic safety. This problem will be considered
later in this chapter.

Methods of Drug Analysis

Analysis for drugs in many ways is more of an art than a
science; there is no harm if different investigators use different methods. However, the results should be in agreement; frequently they are not. Even using the same
method, there may be wide disagreements. In the case of
alcohol, the National Highway Traffic Safety Administra-

tion has arranged a proficiency testing service to improve and standardize the analytical methods. For other drugs, the problem of improvement and standardization of analysis is much more difficult. At present we do not know what is the repeatability within the same laboratory and between different laboratories.

Every technique has inherent limits, and there is a need to recognize and define what is meaningful quantitation. It does not make sense to specify three decimal points if the method is reliable only up to one decimal point. Due to the variation of techniques, confirmation by at least one other method is generally indicated.

In some cases, the blood level of clinical effectiveness is not known, and for none of the drugs has the blood level of performance impairment been established. It may not even be possible to solve this problem of performance impairment. The only significant factor is the brain drug concentration. Even if it was technically feasible, the patient might not like the idea of a brain test. If the blood brain barrier is significant for any particular drug, the blood level will provide too high a value during the ascending phase and too low a value during the descending phase of the blood drug concentration curve. The extent of the problem varies from drug to drug, and it can be solved only by careful analysis of the pharmacodynamics of each individual drug.

A large scale investigation of the pharmacodynamics of drugs and the relation to performance impairment would be justified only if drugs constitute a major safety problem. At present, the data on incidence of drugs in fatally injured drivers are poor, and the incidence figures for other accidents and for drivers on the road are unreliable and difficult to interpret (see Chapter 2).

Some of these studies do not make allowances for differences of annual mileage which can be marked (see Table 22). The question of whether accidents per driver or accidents per 100,000 miles is the appropriate way of expressing a given set of data has to be based on the purpose of the specific study.

Table 22

ANNUAL MILEAGE OF DRUG USERS (15)

Type	Number of Drivers	Licensed Drivers		Unlicensed Drivers	
		Percent	Miles	Percent	Miles
Predrug	743	26	13,900	22	5,760
Nonheroin	780	31	14,000	19	5,945
Heroin	1,500	74	18,300	22	9,200
Methadone	1,470	66	13,950	28	6,000

Another problem with epidemiological drug studies is that it is not possible to compare the incidence for different drugs unless the drugs are compared on a common basis. Some drugs have a high clinical dose. They will be found in body fluids in high concentrations and frequently for days or even weeks after the clinical effect has passed. Other drugs have a low clinical dose. The concentration in body fluids will be low, and it may be difficult to detect them even while they are clinically effective.

There is one obvious, though somewhat crude, way of dealing with this problem, and that is the use of the clinical dose as the common denominator. For instance, a concentration of 1×10^{-5} of the clinical dose per ml of body fluids could be used as a cutoff point. Thus, amphetamine sulfate with a clinical dose of 10 mg would have a cutoff point of 0.1 mc/ml, and pentobarbital sodium with a clinical dose of 100 mg would have a cutoff point of 1 mc/ml. This means that for pentobarbital, all concentrations less than 1 mc/ml are considered negative, while for amphetamine, the sensitivity of detection may have to be increased to assure that concentrations down to 0.1 mc/ml will be detected. In addition, the methods of drug analysis are not standardized. We do not know what the repeatability is within the same laboratory and between different laboratories.

Then there is the question of drugs found in urine or bile. Usually, this could not be considered as an indication that the subject was under the influence of the drug at the time of the accident. However, if there is a delay of sampling it may be the only evidence available. Most of the published studies did not control these factors adequately, and results have to be taken with caution. However, the problems are such that it is doubtful whether we will even have satisfactory information. Therefore, we might as well take the existing information and see what the indications are.

Narcotic Drugs

The public has a strong feeling against the combination of narcotic drugs and driving, and this is reflected in the legal situation. The "Uniform Vehicle Code" (Section 11-902.1) states, "It is unlawful and punishable as provided in Section 11.902.2 for any person who is a habitual user, or under the influence of any narcotic drug, or who is under the influence of any other drug to a degree which renders him incapable of safely driving a vehicle, to drive a vehicle within this state." This, or similar laws, has been passed by all states. However, these laws are based more on emotion than on facts and reason. First, there was not, and there still is no good evidence that driving under the influence of a narcotic drug constitutes a significant safety hazard. Second, there is no way of implementing the law because there is no way of defining what constitutes "under the influence of drugs" and still less what constitutes "under the influence to a degree which renders a person incapable of safe driving."

If we try to define the problem, the first question is, do people drive when under the influence of narcotic drugs? Table 23 shows that there is a good deal of such driving, and these people have to be considered as being under the influence of drugs all the time. They are not under the influence only if they are unable to obtain the drugs, and then they are nervous and jittery and more of a hazard than they are when under the influence. If there should be any need for legal action, it should be directed against the user of narcotic drugs whether under the influence or not.

Table 23 also indicates that much of the driving is done during the day and on weekdays. This differentiates the user of narcotic drugs from the alcoholic. If there is any significant impact on accidents, it is likely to be on non-fatal (daytime) accidents. The following presents a short survey of the evidence of accident involvement.

In 1971, when the Department of Transportation was first confronted with the drug-driving problem, they initiated a review of the literature. This review, by J. L. Nichols of the University of Wisconsin, came to the conclusion that there is no valid evidence that drug use or drug abuse is contributing disproportionately to highway crashes (45).

In the absence of adequate evidence it is surely wrong to assume that there is a safety hazard, but it would have been presumptious to assume that there was no hazard. Therefore, the first government sponsored study was launched in June 1971 (36) to determine the incidence of drugs in fatally injured drivers. Incidence studies are of value only as an indication of a possible problem. If the incidence of drugs in the accident population is low, there is no major safety problem. If the incidence is high, there is a problem only if the incidence in drivers on the road is significantly lower.

Table 23

SUMMARY OF DRIVING FREQUENCY (PERCENT) (15)

	Period		
	Predrug	Heroin	Methadone
Frequency of Driving			
Several times a day	52	69	56
Once a day	9	7	6
Several times a week	22	15	17
Once a week or less	17	9	21
Days of Most Driving			
Weekday	28	22	39
Weekend	36	13	25
About the same	36	64	34
Time Period of Most Driving			
Morning	1	1	1
Daytime	36	31	48
Evening	7	4	4
Morning and evening	10	12	11
Night	25	19	14
Other	21	32	20

NOTE: Percents in this table do not necessarily add to 100 due to rounding.

It is unfortunate that the major Government studies are all on fatal accidents. A negative finding in fatal accidents does not eliminate the possibility of a significant problem in nonfatal accidents. The results of the first study indicated a total drug incidence of 15.2 percent (36) which was considered indicative of a possible safety problem, and it was decided to continue the investigations.

In 1971, the Institute for Research in Public Safety (Indiana University) prepared a "Study of Possible Influences of Licit and Illicit Drugs on Driver Behavior." (24) The study covered 125 subjects and the major conclusions were as follows:

1. There is no evidence that subjects involved in traffic accidents have a greater proportion of drug-positive blood samples than a matched control group.

2. Usage of licit and illicit drugs is statistically unrelated to the number of traffic accidents and moving violations.

3. Accidents and moving violations are more strongly and consistently related to driving history, psychological, and demographic factors than to drug use factors.

In 1972, the Research Triangle Institute, under a combined contract with the Bureau of Narcotics and Dangerous Drugs and the NHTSA (53) examined the criminal, drug, and driving records of 2,270 subjects who had been arrested for various criminal offenses. Of these subjects, 68 percent used some drug at some time for nonmedical reasons. Of those arrested for other reasons than drugs, 50 percent indicated use of drugs. Table 24 shows marked differences in accidents per driver in different parts of the states. However, the data for the control group show that these are due to different standards and methods of reporting, and there is no evidence that they are related to drug use. The rate of convictions (Table 25) is fairly consistent and apparently not related to drug use.

On the whole, the R.T.I. study does not show any significant effect of drugs. However, this is a select group, the variability of the methods is marked, and the number of subjects is limited. The study gained significance, however, when it was confirmed by an investigation that used a completely different approach.

In 1972, Dunlap and Associates, under contract with NHTSA, interviewed, 1,562 methadone maintenance subjects in New York State (15). A control group of 1,059 subjects was matched for age, sex, and socioeconomic background. Complete driving records were obtained for the

Table 24

ACCIDENTS OF SUBJECTS WHO USED NONHEROIN DRUGS BEFORE
DRIVING COMPARED WITH SUBJECTS WHO REPORTED THAT
THEY DID NOT DRIVE IMMEDIATELY AFTER DRUG USE
(PERCENT SUBJECTS WITH ACCIDENTS) (52)

Type	Driving After Drug Use		Not Driving After Drug Use	
	Number	Percent	Number	Percent
Marihuana	671	21.0	67	10.4
Hallucinogens	245	26.9	140	19.3
Amphetamines	373	27.3	65	16.9
Barbiturates	370	28.6	98	12.2
Cocaine	291	25.1	79	19.0
Deliriants	64	28.1	118	17.8
Unspecified	51	27.5	83	36.8
Any Nonheroin drugs*	719	21.0	61	8.1

*Due to multiple usage, this number is less than the sum of the subgroups.

period prior to any drug use, for the period of use of
nonnarcotic drugs (as applicable), for the heroin period,
and for the methadone maintenance time. These data were
obtained for 718 experimental subjects and 579 controls.
The annual mileage is average except for the heroin period when they drive about 50 percent above average, apparently largely to obtain the drugs. Tables 26 and 27
show that the number of violations and accidents is higher
for those who drive immediately after drug use as compared to subjects, who, according to their own statements,
did not drive after drug use. However, there is a marked
difference between the two groups in nonmoving violations (Table 28). Heroin appears to have little effect as far
as the perception of impairment is concerned. They may
be more drowsy (Table 29), but their main concern is not

Table 25

VIOLATIONS OF SUBJECTS WHO USED NONHEROIN DRUGS
BEFORE DRIVING COMPARED WITH SUBJECTS WHO REPORTED
THAT THEY DID NOT DRIVE IMMEDIATELY AFTER DRUG USE
(PERCENT SUBJECTS WITH VIOLATIONS) (52)

Type	Driving After Drug Use		Not Driving After Drug Use	
	Number	Percent	Number	Percent
Marihuana	671	23.8	67	9.0
Hallucinogens	245	29.8	140	21.4
Amphetamines	373	28.7	65	20.0
Barbiturates	370	28.9	98	16.3
Cocaine	291	26.1	79	15.2
Deliriants	64	32.8	118	18.7
Unspecified	51	25.5	83	28.9
Any Nonspecified Drug*	719	23.8	61	8.2

*Due to multiple usage, this number is less than the sum of the subgroups.

being caught by the police (Table 30).

The Dunlap findings on methadone were confirmed by Babst (2) who studied the driving records of 1,576 methadone users and found no difference from the driving records of the average New York driver. Therefore, from a traffic safety point of view, there is no objection to letting methadone users drive.

A recent study by the South Carolina Commission on Alcohol and Drug Abuse (57) indicates that driving after drug use may lead to traffic violations and accidents (Table 31). This study is a controlled study as it compares drug users who drive after drug use with drug users who do not drive after drug use. However, this does not exclude the possibility that there may be other differences between the two groups. Those who drive may include more

Table 26

DISTRIBUTION OF TOTAL TRAFFIC CONVICTIONS 1967-1971
FOR EXPERIMENTAL AND CONTROL GROUPS (15)

Number of Convictions*	Experimental Group		Control Group	
	Number	Percent	Number	Percent
0	370	52	287	50
1	146	20	147	25
2	81	11	74	13
3	56	8	38	7
4	31	4	16	3
5	21	3	10	2
6 or more	13	2	7	1
TOTAL	718		579	

*Excludes equipment and documentation convictions.

chronic users or more people with severe medical disturbances.

Conclusion

Drugs are abused to obtain some effect on the central nervous system. It is not only logical but it can be demonstrated under laboratory conditions that this involves impairment of driving performance. The degree and the nature of impairment may vary. With marihuana it is impaired visual perception and vigilence; with CNS depressant drugs it is attention; and with CNS stimulants it is the ability to concentrate. With narcotic analgesic agents there are some visual hallucinations and possibly perceptual disturbances. However, statistical evidence of an increased involvement in accidents is available only for

Table 27

DISTRIBUTION OF ACCIDENTS (15)

Number of Accidents	Experimental Group		Control Group	
	Number	Percent	Number	Percent
0	399	56	328	57
1	187	26	159	27
2	78	11	67	12
3	34	5	17	3
4	14	2	5	1
5 or more	6	1	3	—
TOTAL	718		579	

Table 28

REVOCATIONS, SUSPENSIONS, AND ADMINISTRATIVE ACTIONS
FOR EXPERIMENTAL AND CONTROL GROUPS (15)

	Experimental Rate Per Driver	Control Rate Per Driver
License Revocations	.11*	.05
License Suspensions	.49	.20
Administrative Actions	1.19	.60
Number	718	579

*Entries are rate per driver summed across five-year period.

alcohol. We have laws prohibiting driving when under the influence of drugs that impair driving performance, and the deterrent effect of these laws may be sufficient to in-

Table 29

MAJOR DIFFERENCE NOTICED IN DRIVING
AFTER HEROIN USAGE (15)

Difference	Percent Citing as Major Difference
No difference	40
Lack of concentration	7
Driving less of a hassle	6
Ability to judge speed impaired	1
Ability to judge distance impaired	1
Ability to judge time impaired	1
Vision problems (including hallucinations)	1
Turned on by driving	2
Nodding out — excessively drowsy	22
Drove better	9
Weaving, reckless driving	—
Indecisiveness in reacting to emergency situations	1
Nervous, defensive	3
Lack of physical coordination	4
Other	4
No answer	1

duce drug abusers to drive with such care that their driving record is not worse than that of a driver without drugs.

From a traffic safety point of view, the only significant factor is whether there is any effect on accidents, and obviously there is no evidence of any significant effect. However, we cannot say that the laws prohibiting driving while under the influence of these drugs are wrong. The Dunlap study (Table 32) indicates that the law may be a very important factor controlling the driving behavior of this group. Any change of the law, a change of the drug usage pattern, or of the public attitude towards drug abuse

Table 30

MAIN THING ON MIND OF HEROIN USER WHILE DRIVING
IMMEDIATELY AFTER USING HEROIN (15)

Main Thing on Mind	Percent
Driving well enough to avoid being stopped by the police	36
Enjoying the high	18
Not caring about anything	11
Fear of accident	7
Fear of getting stopped	7
Not driving well	2
Physical discomfort	1
Other	12
No response	5

may upset the situation. There is no need for any active steps at this time, but there is a need for periodic reevaluation of this situation.

Marihuana

According to current estimates, some 36 million people in this country have tried marihuana, and about 15 million people have used it within the last month. A breakdown of the usage pattern is presented in Table 32.

Under laboratory conditions, a number of reports indicate impairment of the detection of visual and auditory signals, difficulty of concentrating and of making quick decision, and a slower response time resulting in impaired performance of some manipulative tasks and in muscular coordination among users of marihuana. Klonoff (31) examined the effect of marihuana under controlled conditions when driving on a driving course and on city streets.

Table 31

DRUGS AND DRIVING

	OTC Drugs		Prescription Drugs		Illicit Drugs	
	Drive	No Drive	Drive	No Drive	Drive	No Drive
At least 1 ticket/ 3 years	37	28	35	32	57	31
At least 1 accident/3 years	28	25	30	24	26	25

NOTE: Figures are percent.
The study compares people who report driving after drug use with those who maintain that they do not drive after use.

Table 32

AGE AND SEX DISTRIBUTION OF MARIHUANA USE (41)

		Age			Sex	
	Mean	18-25	26-34	35+	M	F
Percent ever Used	21	53	36	6	29	14
Percent Current Use	8	25	11	1	11	5

Marihuana tends to induce impairment of judgment, care, and concentration. About one-third of the smokers showed no significant change, and one-fourth showed significant improvement of performance.

The main active ingredient, tertrahydrocannabinol, reaches a peak concentration in the blood in about ten minutes. The concentration comes down to 5 percent within one hour, but the impairment effects can last for many hours. However, the laboratory impairment does not necessarily mean that there is a traffic safety problem. Even Klonoff's findings indicate impairment and not necessarily a safety hazard (31). If the driver is aware of the impairment, he (she) may be able to compensate. A driver who is under the influence of alcohol is likely to drive fast and recklessly, but if you ask a marihuana smoker whether he drives when under the influence of marihuana, the typical response is, "Are you kidding?" Actually, they do drive, but being aware of the impairment and possibly due to some distortion of time perception, they tend to drive slowly. Frequently, they complain about other drivers passing them. "I drove at maximum speed and everybody was passing me." The awareness of performance impairment of the marihuana smoker is well presented by Sterling Smith (58) in Table 33, but even an impaired marihuana smoker is not a greater traffic hazard than the normal driver if he can compensate for the impairment.

The only meaningful evidence of a safety hazard would be epidemiological data comparing the marihuana smoker with a suitable control group, and this evidence is not available. In 1972, when we had no chemical tests for the identification of marihuana in body fluids, we had a marihuana symposium (4) and I made the following statement: "Preliminary evidence indicates that marihuana impairs the ability to drive. However, marihuana apparently is not a significant factor in the statistical incidence of fatal and non-fatal accidents. These two observations, if combined, indicate that either the marihuana smoker is conscious of the impairment and avoids driving, or that he manages to compensate for the deficiency, at least to some extent." Now we do have reliable tests for the quantitative identification of marihuana in body fluids, and the 1972 statement still holds true. This does not mean that it is correct,

Table 33

OPERATORS' SELF-EVALUATION REGARDING DRIVING
ABILITIES WHEN UNDER THE INFLUENCE OF MARIHUANA (58)

Driving Evaluation	Marihuana Smoking Patterns			TOTAL
	Light	Moderate	Heavy	
Drive Better	2 (18%)	4 (5%)	14 (10%)	20 (8%)
Drive the same	4 (37%)	31 (37%)	56 (38%)	91 (38%)
Drive worse	5 (45%)	49 (58%)	77 (52%)	131 (54%)
TOTAL	11 (100%)	84 (100%)	147 (100%)	242 (100%)

but it is difficult to obtain the kind of information that would confirm or refute the concept. Ethical principles of protection of the public do not allow stopping a driver on the road and requesting a blood sample.

Some evidence of a possible hazard comes from Sterling Smith's study (Table 34). The differences in this study are comparatively small. The identification of marihuana smokers was based on interviews, not on actual analysis; therefore, the data cannot be considered as good evidence of a marihuana problem, and in the absence of adequate evidence the public is divided as to the safety and the need of countermeasures. The marihuana users are against any kind of control as shown in Table 35, and from the legal point of view, driving while under the influence of marihuana is unlawful. Obviously, there is an urgent need of getting the information and settling the problem.

Table 34

INVOLVEMENT OF MARIHUANA SMOKER
IN FATAL ACCIDENTS (58)

| | Smoker | | Nonsmoker | |
	Number	Percent	Number	Percent
Fatal Accidents	121	45	146	55
Control	272	34	529	66

The following outlines the kind of study that could be done even with current restrictions. There are major marihuana centers in most bigger towns as well as in major universities. We could take a sample of marihuana smokers from several centers, ask each smoker to give the name of a friend who is the same age, the same sex, and the same socioeconomic background and who is *not* on marihuana. Then we collect and compare the driving records for the smokers and the controls. If there is no difference between the two groups, it is a good indication that marihuana does not present a significant traffic safety hazard. If there is a difference, it identifies the marihuana smokers as a high risk group, but this does not necessarily mean that the risk was due to marihuana. There could be some psychological factor that is likely to lead to marihuana smoking as well as to greater accident involvement.

Nicotine

The most interesting result of the studies by the Midwest Research Institute (36,37) may be the marked risk factor for nicotine in the blood (9.66) as compared with the low factor (1.2) when the urinary findings are added (Table

Table 35

ATTITUDES TOWARD MARIHUANA AND
VEHICLE OPERATION (30)

Group (By Use)	Number	Percentage of Group Against Vehicle Operation Under the Influence of Marihuana		
		Airplane Pilots	Taxicab Drivers	Private Drivers
Nonusers*	247	92%	89%	91%
Nonusers†	16	94%	94%	79%
Former Users	72	92%	87%	77%
Infrequent Users	38	76%	54%	50%
Weekly Users	46	84%	59%	24%
Chronic Users	100	67%	38%	21%

*This Nonuser group includes those who have never witnessed a driver under the influence of marihuana.
†This group includes only those Nonusers who have witnessed a driver under the influence of marihuana.

36). The risk factor for all drugs in the blood is 3.54. If it had been heroin instead of nicotine, it would have hit the national and possibly even the international newsstands. As it was nicotine, it was bypassed. It did not fit the pattern of "hazardous drugs," therefore, it had to be an artifact. Actually, the evidence is very strong, and there is no justification to neglect it. However, the evidence does not necessarily mean that this is a pharmacological risk.

There is a good indication of a high risk group, and there is good evidence that these people did smoke shortly before the accident. We do not know whether the nicotine had anything to do with the accident. It could be that smoking while driving is an indication of extreme nervousness which is likely to cause accidents, or it could be that the mechanical factor of smoking while driving inter-

Table 36

NICOTINE IN BLOOD AND FATAL ACCIDENTS (36,37)

	Fatal			Control			Risk Factor
	Total Number	Nicotine Number	Percent	Total Number	Nicotine Number	Percent	
MRI 1974	682	57	8.4	977	19	1.94	4.33
MRI 1975	825	113	13.7	817	2	0.24	57.1
TOTAL	1507	170	11.3	1794	21	1.17	9.66

feres with the efficiency of car control. Anyway, we have here a high risk group where the incidence is about as great as all drugs combined and the risk factor is greater than any individual drug or any group of drugs. In addition, this is a group where corrective action may be easier than it is for other drugs, but nothing has been done or is being done, and even the public has not been informed of the observations.

Chapter 6

DRUGS AND MEDICAL IMPAIRMENT

CLINICAL ASPECTS

MOST drivers who have a chronic medical condition and many drivers with acute medical conditions do take therapeutic drugs. If the medical condition impairs driving performance and decreases the accident survival rate, the therapeutic effect of the drugs is likely to reduce the medical hazard. However, the drugs may also have side effects that may cause impairment of driving performance. Therefore, as far as accident survival rate is concerned, the effect of drugs is likely to be beneficial; as far as driving performance is concerned, the effect may be beneficial or harmful. Most of the existing literature considers medical impairment or drugs, while actually the two cannot be separated.

The following presents a short survey of some of the major medical conditions that can affect driving performance with emphasis on the degree to which the safety hazard is modified by the use of drugs. Unfortunately, such a discussion has to be vague. We realize that there should be definite standards for people who want to drive a private car, a cargo transport, or a passenger transport, but we have no objective standards. Medical Boards generally make their decision on a clinical basis that may have little relevance to the actual driving performance. We might be able to develop a test of driving capability, but generally people with chronic medical conditions drive very little and they are usually cautious. In addition, being able to drive is an extremely important economic as well as emotional factor. If we deal with alcohol or drug abuse,

71

there is a certain correction potential. In medically induced impairment, the subject is completely innocent, and the correction potential may be very low. Therefore, the question should not be whether or not to get a license, but what can be done to decrease the safety hazard to such an extent that a subject may be able to drive without undue danger to the rest of the driving population.

The government is, and has to be, interested in traffic safety. Trying to use legal restrictions, you work against people; trying to decrease the hazard by creation of an optimal driving condition makes it possible to work with the people and with maximal public support. So far, the emphasis has been on enforcement, arrest, and legal limits. It has not worked. After eight years of research in drugs and driving, we have not come up with anything that even looks as if it might become an effective countermeasure. On the other hand, we can use drugs to improve traffic safety. If someone has a severe cold, he needs some assistance to be able to safely operate a motor vehicle. To tell such a person, "Do not drive after the use of antihistamines," may protect the manufacturer and the government, but it does not help the driver. As mentioned before, driving is an important economic, social, and emotional factor, and our person with a severe cold is likely to drive anyway. Therefore, it should be the task of the government to provide the information that optimizes this person's driving capability. We should provide information as to when antihistamines are indicated and when they should be avoided. Out of the twenty possible antihistamines, which ones are the most suitable from the driving point of view (maximum therapeutic effects with minimal side effects); what is the appropriate dose, and how often should the drug be taken? The same kind of information is required for people with hypertension, diabetes, migraine headaches, allergies, and for the 20 million people who use tranquilizers.

Much of the required information is available now, or it can be developed fairly easily. We can determine when to use antihistamines and which antihistamines to use without knowing what is the safety hazard of a cold, what is the hazard of an antihistamine in a healthy person, and what is the hazard of a person with a cold under various kinds of treatments. If we wanted to obtain all this information first, it would take many years and would have little effect on the information we would finally provide to the sick driver. Drawing upon eight years of research in the drug-driving area did not contribute anything to the solution of this problem, and if we continue the same way for another eight years, we will probably not be any further along.

The following is a short survey of the major areas where we have the problem of drug-health interaction.

Epilepsy

Epilepsy is actually not a disease but a symptom. Essentially, it refers to a lowering of the seizure threshold, which may be congenital or it may be due to a variety of causes, such as trauma, tumor, inflammation, or alcoholism. Since attacks, involving lapses of consciousness, can occur without definable provocation, uncontrolled epilepsy presents a major driving hazard. A serious condition is the grand mal, but from the driving point of view it may be less of a hazard, because the grand mal attacks are usually preceded by an aura. However, any attack that includes symptoms such as involuntary running, fighting, and convulsions could constitute such a safety hazard that no patient should be allowed to drive unless the condition is fully controlled by drugs, such as phenobarbitone or diphenylhydantoin. These drugs do impair driving performance, but the dosage required for clinical control of epilepsy is comparatively low, and the patients are well adapted to the drug. Therefore, we have here a condition where even a conservative body, such as the American Medical Association, recommends that the patient whose condition is adequately controlled by drugs should be allowed to drive.

Mental Illness

Major tranquilizers (antipsychotic drugs) that are used to control abnormal thoughts and behavior have marked sedative and muscular side effects, but even when the clinical condition is adequately controlled by drugs, these people cannot be considered safe drivers.

Depression

Tricyclic compounds, MAO inhibitors, and lithium carbonate may provide a reasonable control of the clinical condition, but there are only very few cases where conditions are such that driving can even be considered.

Anxiety

Without drugs, anxiety presents a safety hazard (driver is jittery, likely to overcompensate and overreact). Drugs are likely to be beneficial, but the condition is so poorly defined that no meaningful data are available. If handled by a physician, the use of sedatives and tranquilizers may control the condition adequately. If the use of the same drugs is left to the patient, it is more likely to constitute a hazard, especially at night.

Cardiovascular Disease

Very few of these subjects do not use drugs (digitalis in congestive heart failure, vascular relaxants in hypertension). The main problems are with lapse of consciousness and lower accident survival rate. Both are improved by the use of drugs. Even with drugs, driving should be allowed only in mild cases under well-controlled conditions.

Diabetes

Uncontrolled diabetes can be a safety hazard affecting driving performance as well as the accident survival rate. The same applies to overmedication, i.e. the hypergly-cemic response to insulin. However, there is no reason why a well-controlled diabetic subject should not drive. This is another condition where the use of drugs may be a prerequisite for driving.

Arthritis

Untreated arthritis may interfere with the mechanical part of driving performance. Salicylates and corticosteroids may facilitate driving, and these drugs have no negative effects on driving performance. However, the use of muscle relaxants and curarelike agents should be considered hazardous, at least for the first 48 hours after use.

Parkinson's Disease

The disease may interfere with driving performance, and symptomatic relief by agents such as levodopa and belladonna may facilitate driving. Issuance of a driving permit should be based on a careful evaluation of the specific case.

Narcolepsy

This is an obvious case where an untreated patient is a traffic hazard, and the use of drugs (stimulants) improves performance. Unfortunately, there is little information available as to the extent of impairment, what tests should be used, and what constitutes adequate control. The absence of reliable criteria makes it difficult to justify the issuance of a driving permit.

Migraine

A patient with an untreated migraine would constitute a safety problem, but he (she) is not likely to drive anyway. Treatment with drugs such as ergot would facilitate driving, but there are no objective criteria that indicate if and when driving should be permitted.

Cold

A cold can cause a serious impairment of driving performance. Drug therapy (antihistamines) will improve the signs and symptoms of the cold, but the side effects may constitute as much of a hazard as the original cold. If driving cannot be avoided, only a physician may be able to advise whether in the specific case a drug should or should not be used.

These are just a few examples indicating that there is such a close interrelationship between drugs and impaired health as to affect driving performance, as well as the accident survival rate. In some cases, the evidence of impairment is clearcut, and definite rules can be established. For instance, in epilepsy, the presence or absence of attacks is a matter of fact and can be used to establish rules as to the adequacy of control by drugs; the American Medical Association recommends that subjects be allowed to drive if they are free of seizures for at least two years. However, in most cases, the possibility and the degree of impairment are difficult to define, and in such cases, it has to be left to Medical Boards to determine, on a case-by-case basis, whether driving can be permitted.

This survey leads to one important conclusion, and that is that under a variety of conditions, the use of properly prescribed therapeutic drugs improves driving performance and accident survival rate. These people are probably more of a safety hazard than the average healthy driver even when the clinical symptoms are controlled by drugs, however, the hazard would be greater without the drugs.

A problem arises with the drugs, such as the tranquilizers where we have some 20 million users and very few who use them on a strictly medical basis. Mostly, these drugs are taken because the patient believes that it will make him (her) feel better. Under these conditions, these are drugs of abuse similar to alcohol and marihuana. The main difference is probably that alcohol and marihuana are frequently taken to the point where they cause marked performance impairment and the tranquilizers to the point of relief of tension, which may or may not be accompanied by impaired driving performance. In view of the magnitude of the possible problem, there is a need to determine the nature and extent of performance impairment, and this will be discussed in a following section of this chapter.

EPIDEMIOLOGICAL ASPECTS

Under laboratory conditions, psychoactive drugs impair driving performance. This has been demonstrated again and again. Unfortunately, this has very little application to the real traffic safety problem. If you take a normal, healthy subject and give him (her) a psychoactive drug, it would be surprising if there was no performance impairment. But if the same drug is used for legitimate medical purposes, it is intended to correct or compensate for an existing deficiency. Performance was probably impaired before the drug was taken, and it may still be impaired when the drug becomes effective, but most likely there is some improvement. A typical example are eyeglasses. Giving properly prescribed glasses to a shortsighted person is likely to improve his driving performance, but giving the same glasses to a person with normal eyesight would impair his driving performance.

As a general rule, it can be stated that if a medical condition is associated with marked performance impairment, therapeutic drugs are likely to improve performance; if there is little performance impairment, the use of therapeutic drugs before driving should be avoided. The question is then, which are the conditions that are likely to cause accidents? Since performance impairment data do not indicate how far a person can compensate for the deficiency, the most meaningful information comes from the epidemiological studies.

Table 37 is taken from the Statistical Abstracts, 1976 (63) and shows that limitations of activity due to chronic diseases is a fairly common phenomenon. The last line, "Total," is derived by addition of the other number, which neglects the possibility of overlap. On the other hand, the table does not include acute conditions and injuries. Therefore, it may be a crude indication of the extent of medically induced limitation of activity. Table 38 indicates that drivers who are officially certified as medically impaired are overrepresented in property damage accidents, and Table 39 shows that the degree of overrepresentation is even more pronounced for injury accidents. No equivalent for fatal accidents was available, though the data from the Virginia Highway Research Council (Table 40) indicate a comparatively low ratio of the observed incidence over the expected incidence.

There are a number of factors to be considered in the interpretation of these data. First, the data are expressed in terms of accidents per 100 million miles, and medically impaired drivers generally drive very little. If the data were

Table 37

PERSONS WITH ACTIVITY LIMITATIONS BY SELECTED CHRONIC CONDITIONS (63)

(%)

	Both Sexes		Males				Females			
	All Ages	65+	All Ages	-45	45-64	65+	All Ages	-45	45-64	65+
Heart Conditions	13.4	18.8	13.8	4.4	18.7	19.2	13.1	5.9	13.4	18.5
Arthritis, Rheumatism	11.2	16.9	7.5	2.3	9.2	11.6	15.0	4.7	16.9	21.3
Hypertension	2.9	4.0	1.8	0.8	2.0	2.8	3.9	2.0	4.4	4.9
Mental and Nervous Disorder	3.7	1.7	3.5	5.0	4.0	1.3	3.8	4.9	4.7	2.1
TOTAL	31.2	41.4	26.6	12.5	33.9	34.9	35.8	17.5	39.4	46.8

Table 38

ACCIDENT INVOLVEMENT OF MEDICALLY IMPAIRED GROUP (42)

| Number of Accidents | Property Damage Accidents (%) | | Ratio |
	Medical Group*	Control	
1	26.06	19.34	1.35
2	12.54	5.25	2.39
3	11.40	3.23	3.51

*24,992 medically impaired drivers; 3,311,720 controls.

Table 39

ACCIDENT INVOLVEMENT OF MEDICALLY IMPAIRED GROUP (42)

| Number of Accidents | Injury Accidents* (%) | | Ratio |
	Medical Group†	Control	
1	16.38	6.59	2.49
2	3.59	0.75	˙4.79
3	1.03	0.15	6.86

*Driver record (including fatal accidents).
†24,992 medically impaired drivers; 3,311,720 controls.

expressed in terms of accidents per driver, the ratio would be considerably higher. Actually, we would expect a marked effect of medical impairment on fatal accidents due to the low accident survival rate. On the other hand, medically impaired people generally drive slowly, and they are more likely to drive during the day, while fatal accidents occur primarily at night (see Table 8).

Table 40

FATAL ACCIDENTS OF DRIVERS WITH CHRONIC
MEDICAL CONDITIONS* (64)

Condition	Expected	Observed	Ratio
Epilepsy	8.2	16.0	1.95
Cardiovascular Disease	9.0	14.6	1.62
Diabetes	8.7	15.5	1.78
Alcoholism	6.8	11.3	1.66
Mental Illness	7.2	15.3	2.13
Drug Use	6.8	11.3	1.66
Miscellaneous	7.4	20.7	2.79

*Fatal crashes per 100 million miles.
†2,675 subjects with chronic medical conditions and 926 controls.

A theoretical analysis (Table 41) indicates that medical impairment may have a greater effect on the accident survival rate than on driving performance. This is important because in earlier studies the effect of drugs on the accident survival rate had been completely neglected. Table 42 shows that the group of medically impaired drivers has a marked increase in multiple convictions for reckless driving. The fact that in nonmoving violations (Table 43) there is little evidence of a significant effect of medical impairment may be an indication that the convictions for reckless driving might be due to physical limitations, such as impaired visual performance or prolonged response time, rather than the psychological attitude of recklessness.

The risk factor used in medical impairment is based on a different approach and cannot be compared with the risk factor in controlled alcohol and drug studies. When evaluating a drug, we have a condition, and the ideal method is comparing the same subject with and without the drug.

Table 41

MAJOR MEDICAL DISABILITIES AND DRIVING HAZARDS
(24,992 DRIVERS) (42)

Condition	Percent	Performance Impairment*	Lower Accident Survival Rate*
Hypertension	1.86	—	1.86
Coronary Artery Diseases	16.29	—	16.29
Valvular Heart Disease	1.30	—	1.30
Cerebrovascular Accident	4.40	—	4.40
Cardiac Arrhythmias	0.62	—	0.62
Congestive Heart Failure	2.23	—	2.23
Diabetes	3.53	1.77	3.53
Epilepsy	11.61	5.81	
Other Neurological Conditions	2.46	2.46	
Paralysis	0.74	0.74	
Arthritis	1.09	1.09	
Bone and Muscular Disturbances	0.84	0.84	
Visual Disturbances	5.38	5.38	
Mental Illness	15.82	—	
Alcoholism	20.52	10.26†	20.52
TOTAL		30.31	50.75

*Author's interpretation.
†Only when intoxicated.

In the case of medical impairment, we deal with people where the condition cannot be separated from the person. The risk is determined by comparing the experimental group with a matched control group. Place of an accident, day of the week, and time of day are generally not important parameters for a control. Age may be important, but that depends on the nature of the disturbance. Mental illness strikes all people of all ages while cardiovascular diseases are largely limited to older people. Therefore, if you do not control for age, it will have little effect on the risk factor for mental disturbances, and it will markedly

Table 42

CONVICTIONS FOR RECKLESS DRIVING — DRIVERS WITH
MEDICAL RECORDS AND CONTROLS (42)

Convictions	Medical Record*	Control	Ratio
None	85.78%	95.66	0.90
1	9.89	3.33	2.97
2	2.94	0.63	4.67
3	0.94	0.16	5.88
4+	0.42	0.02	21.00

*24,992 medically impaired drivers; 3,311,720 controls.

Table 43

NONMOVING VIOLATION RATES FOR DRIVERS WITH CHRONIC
MEDICAL CONDITIONS* (64)

Condition	Expected†	Observed	O/E Ratio
Epilepsy	3.4	4.7	1.38
Cardiovascular Disease	2.7	3.6	1.34
Diabetes	3.3	4.6	1.39
Alcoholism	2.5	4.6	1.84
Mental Illness	3.0	5.3	1.77
Drug Use	3.6	6.4	1.78
Miscellaneous	2.8	4.9	1.75

*Citations per 100,000 miles.
†2,675 subjects with chronic medical conditions and 926 controls.

increase the risk factor for cardiovascular disturbances.
The same applies to drug treatment. If a drug is used for
the treatment of cardiovascular disease (tranquilizer), con-

trol for the age factor is essential. If the same drug is used for the treatment of emotional disturbances, the control for age is of no importance.

PERFORMANCE, ACCIDENTS

The effect of medical impairment, with and without drugs, on performance and accidents is discussed in a number of studies. Haddon (19) found in 1961 that in pedestrian accidents, the fatally injured drivers were about 10 years older than the survivors. Smith (56) in 1968 reported that 10 to 20 percent of the driving population are taking prescribed drugs at any point in time. In addition, drugs are being used unauthorized. But there is no evidence that drug users are overrepresented in accidents. Baker and Spitz (3) in 1970 stated that "the decreased ability to survive crashes caused older persons to be greatly overrepresented among fatally injured drivers. The proportion of drivers who were 60 years of age or older was 5 times as high among those killed as among those who survived multiple vehicle crashes." Kibrik and Smart maintained that 3 to 5 percent of the driving population are taking prescribed drugs (29) and 11 to 15 percent of the accident involved drivers have taken psychoactive drugs prior to the accident. Waller (66) gives a good review of the evidence for medically induced impairment of driving performance, but there is little evidence that the impairment may have been modified by the use of drugs. Legg (32), in 1973, using amobarbital and nitrazapam, found impairment of cognitive and motor performance in normal subjects and no impairment in anxious subjects. Hollister (21) comes to similar conclusions: "The net effect of psychotherapeutic drugs may be beneficial rather than harmful. Unrelieved anxiety, depression, or psychosis may be a greater threat to traffic safety than any possible adverse effect of the drug on performance." A report of the

Oregon State Board of Health (46) lists the following as the leading medical causes of driving impairment:

Cardiac and Circulatory Disturbance	36.7 percent
Lapse of Consciousness	14.2 "
Epilepsy	14.0 "
Diabetes	10.0 "
Neurological Disorders	4.7 "
Cerebro-vascular Accidents	3.8 "
Others	16.6 "

This survey of the literature is incomplete, but it indicates the problem. There is not a single study that provides adequate information on medical as well as drug aspects of the problem, though this would have been possible in most of these investigations. There is not a single well-controlled study, and (as discussed in Chapter 2) it would be very difficult, if not impossible, to obtain a meaningful risk factor for the various drugs.

Finally, the findings of most of these studies are bounded by the limits of the methods of analysis, and this is something that is not a major obstacle anymore.

The most interesting information comes from a 1975 study by the Midwest Research Institute (37). This study compares the incidence of drugs in fatally injured drivers with the incidence in drivers on the road. As in all drug studies, it is easy to find problems: inadequate participation of drivers on the road, inadequate medical information, and inadequate analytical techniques. These limitations should be considered when interpreting the results, but they should not be taken as reason to reject the whole study. The data presented in Table 44 are considered acceptable because any error of the study would apply equally to the two groups that are being compared. According to the data presented in Table 44, the risk factor for drugs in trace amounts (less than 1 mc/l) is greater than it is for drugs in levels of possible performance impairment (greater than 1 mc/1). If a drug is present in trace amounts, this is considered an indication of a drug user who was not under the influence of drugs at the time of the accident. Therefore, the data do indicate that in the drug user population, drugs may decrease the risk factor or at least, the use of drugs does not increase the risk factor. Most surveys — Perrine, 1975 (48), Clayton, 1976 (13), Willette, 1977 (68), and Jocelyn (26) — are essentially in agreement that there is no good evidence that therapeutic drugs are a traffic safety hazard.

Table 44

DRUG INCIDENCE IN LIVING AND FATALLY
INJURED DRIVERS (37)

| | Drug Level of Possible Impairment* | | Drugs in Trace Amounts† | |
	Living Drivers	Fatally Injured	Living Drivers	Fatally Injured
Sample Size (No.)	763	503	763	503
Incidence of Drugs (No.)	20	51	12	38
Incidence of Drugs (%)	2.62	10.1	1.57	7.6
Risk Factor (Calculated)	3.85		4.84	

*Drugs in blood at any concentration and/or in urine or bile above 1 mc/ml.
†Blood negative for drugs, and urine and/or bile in concentrations below 1 mc/ml.

Countermeasures

We never had any drug countermeasure campaign, but

the research effort was based on the same misconception we find in the alcohol program.

If someone has a severe cold and has to drive, let us say from Philadelphia to New York, the question arises whether or not to take an antihistamine before driving. The degree of risk varies again according to the difference of impairment before and/or after the use of the countermeasure.

1. If we consider the drug user as his own control, the risk factor will be essentially unaffected by the use of the drug. Some people will be better drivers with the drug, and others will be better drivers without the drug — the net effect can be considered as zero.

2. If another person drives instead of the driver with the cold, the risk would be reduced, say from 4 to 2.

3. If the whole trip was cancelled, the risk would be reduced to zero.

The government sponsored experiments evaluate the risk according to number 2, i.e. comparing the sick driver with a normal healthy driver. But the countermeasures (drug labeling, public education, enforcement) are more likely to lead to a decision as to whether or not to use the drug before driving according to number 1. Therefore, most of the information that has been obtained and is being obtained by current and planned programs is irrelevant to the person who wants to know whether or not to use a drug before driving, as well as to the congressman who wants to know whether drug use before driving should be prohibited.

Therapeutic drugs have a two-sided effect: a therapeutic effect that is beneficial (it tends to increase the accident survival rate and to improve driving performance) and a side effect that is likely to impair driving performance. Obviously, the target of a countermeasure effort has to be the elimination or inhibition of the side effects without interference with the therapeutic effects. A number of ways may be considered to achieve this target:

1. The government can evaluate the ratio of therapeutic-to-side effects for any group of commercially available drug preparations and make the results available to the public, the druggists, and to the medical profession. For instance, if there are twenty antihistamines, the public wants to know which preparations can be used safely before driving.

2. When drugs are administered, the concentration of the drug or of the active metabolites in the blood rises rapidly and then declines at a slower rate (Figure 3). When the drug concentration comes close to the minimum effective concentration, the administration has to be repeated. The extent of side effects is determined by the concentration curve, which means it reaches a minimum shortly before the new dose is applied. If a subject can schedule his (her) driving to coincide with the low part of the concentration curve, he (she) can avoid severe side effects while driving.

3. A more promising approach may be the use of multiple low doses instead of a few high doses (see Figure 3). Instead of taking 40 mg of drug X every 4 hours, the driver may take 10 mg every 90 minutes. The frequent drug ingestion is cumbersome to the patient and the therapeutic effect may not be fully equivalent to the usual method of drug application. But the scheme provides a period of relatively safe driving, and this period can be extended as required.

4. The same goal of a blood-drug concentration just slightly above the minimum effective level could be achieved by a sustained drug release. Multilayer capsules or capsules with tiny pellets can be prepared where breakdown occurs over a given time period as determined by the characteristics of the coating layer. The difficulty is the lack of a suitable depot with constant environmental characteristics. If the capsule could be maintained in the

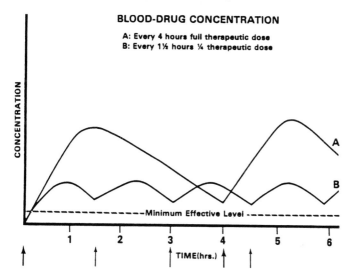

Figure 3: The relationship of drug dose to the blood drug concentration.

mouth or stomach, the method would work. But it is difficult to use such a method if the drug passes through the intestinal tract at an unknown and uncontrollable rate. Implantation works, but it is too traumatic for the vast majority of the cases.

5. It may be possible to increase the ratio of the therapeutic-to-side effects by combination of drugs, where the therapeutic effects are synergistic while the side effects are not. It may also be possible to use a combination where drug B specifically inhibits the side effects of drug A. The government does not have to get involved into the development of such agents, but the government should set up standards that a manufacturer should meet if he wants to advertise that his agent can safely be taken before driving.

The five approaches just discussed represent possible countermeasures that can be explored, developed, and applied at this time without waiting for the results of the extensive and prolonged studies that are being conducted by the government. Actually, the implementation of this kind of countermeasure is not facilitated by anything the government has done in the past or is doing now. Further, it is not clear what other practical countermeasures might result from current government plans and programs.

Chapter 7

DISCUSSION AND CONCLUSIONS

THE following presents discussion, conclusions, and recommendations for those areas that the author considers the major problem areas in the drug-driving field.

The Interaction of Medical Impairment and The Use of Therapeutic Drugs

Medically induced performance impairment and therapeutic drugs should be considered as independent and interrelated variables. You cannot consider the safety risk of a medical condition (performance and accident survival rate) without also considering the degree to which the risk may be modified by the use of therapeutic drugs; and you cannot consider the safety impact of therapeutic drugs without also considering the condition of the driver prior to drug use.

Accident Survival Rate

In people of advanced age and people with chronic diseases, the chances that they will succumb to accidental injuries is increased, and the presence of such a person in an accident may convert an otherwise nonfatal accident into a fatal accident. This factor has largely been neglected in earlier risk evaluation, but it may play a major role in the use of drugs in the prevention of fatal accidents. A driver with severe hypertension has a low accident survival rate, and this condition may be improved with the use of drugs.

The Controlled Drug Study

In the alcohol field, a series of major epidemiological studies were conducted where the control group had restrictions as to time and place that were not imposed on the accident group. This approach greatly limits the usefulness of the resulting data. Nonetheless, the same approach was used in some major drug studies. The impact of such a bias into the drug area varies. If time and place are important parameters, results are essentially useless. If age, sex, and socioeconomic background are more important than time and place, results may be little affected by the bias. For future drug studies, the experimental parameters for each drug have to be carefully selected, and they have to be applied to the accident as well as to the control group.

Decreased Emphasis on Enforcement

In the past, the government's role in traffic safety was considered largely in the area of enforcement, legal limits, and arrest. Gradually it became apparent that this is not a cost-effective approach. The chances of an intoxicated driver being arrested are 1:2,000. This means that an enforcement effort can be effective only as long as the public does not realize how low the chances of a "driving while intoxicated" arrest are. The British alcohol campaign of 1968 was successful because the public grossly overestimated the chances of DWI arrest, and it collapsed when the public became aware of the situation (53). An intensive enforcement effort might increase the chances of arrest to 1:500 or even 1:100. But even with a chance of 1:100, the deterrent effect of enforcement is very low.

Increasing the arrest rate creates the problem as to what to do with the arrestee. If you put him (her) behind bars, this will be for a limited time, and once released, he (she) will probably resume the old drinking pattern.

The difficulties of enforcement are enhanced by the increasing social importance of individual right and freedom. Therefore, it is suggested that the basic government approach be changed and that we try to work with the driver instead of against the driver. The actual approach is largely determined by the extent of the drinking problem.

The Social Drinker

The social drinker is generally amenable to countermeasures. The purpose of a countermeasure effort in traffic safety is somewhat different from the target of an effort by the Department of Health, Education, and Welfare (HEW). In traffic safety, we want to make sure that the person does not drink to the point of impairment or that he does not drive when intoxicated. A punitive approach (Keep the Drunken Driver Off the Streets, He Kills Your Children) is likely to lead to conflicts with HEW where alcoholism is considered a curable disease. But the DOT effort does not have to be in conflict with the HEW effort, and emphasis on the punitive aspects enhances the difficulty of safety education and training.

Social drinkers generally resent government interference, and a DWI arrest is a poor basis for any kind of rehabilitation. DWI laws and enforcement are necessary, but rehabilitation should be part of a separate education and training effort.

Since the legal limits are in terms of the blood alcohol concentration, enforcement has to be based on the BAC concept and test. However, rehabilitation should be based on working with the individual, on alcohol as a disease, and on the concept of individual limits of impairment, which are mostly lower than the legal limits. The BAC and the individual limits of performance impairment are statistically correlated. But there is a wide range of performance impairment for any given BAC. Therefore, when dealing with individual cases, the two approaches cannot be used interchangeably. The BAC test should be used for enforcement, and no performance test should be used in connection with legal and arrest procedures.

In alcohol education and training, we want to make sure that no impaired person drives. Therefore, we should use only tests and concepts of individual performance limits. The concept and test of legal limits should be avoided because it may actually encourage drinking beyond the individual safe driving limits.

The Problem Drinker

In the past, all efforts to rehabilitate problem drinkers had no effect on accidents, or they increased the accident rate. It is not likely that this will change in the future. The problem is alcoholism, and the basic approach is probably primary prevention; this is beyond the scope of a Traffic Safety Administration. The only area where we can reduce the safety hazard is by improving the accident survival rate.

Alcohol Countermeasures

In developing countermeasure programs and in the projection of the benefits of the proposed programs, the impairment of the intoxicated driver is compared with the impairment of the at-risk driver on the road. The results of such studies show a reduction of the safety risk from 20 to 2, however, the actual campaign tries to induce the driver to reduce his alcohol intake from supralegal to sublegal levels. If successful, this reduces the safety risk from 20 to 10. Therefore, the projection indicates a marked reduction of accidents (by a factor of 10) while the actual impact is minimal (factor of 2).

There is a need for a better understanding of the driver and his needs. We have to know who drinks to become intoxicated and who drinks for the taste or for social purposes. For the first group, enforcement may be the appropriate method. For the second group, we should use performance limits instead of legal limits. Further, we may want to prohibit advertising and to increase taxation. We may decide to lower the alcohol concentration of commercial products and to develop means of increasing the breakdown on alcohol in the gastrointestinal tract. We may want to increase the antialcohol drive by determining the cancerogenic effects of alcohol.

Narcotic Drugs

Narcotic analgesic drugs are apparently no significant traffic safety problem at this time, but a change of the law or a change of the public attitude may change the situation.

Marihuana

The possible safety hazard of marihuana has not been determined. There is a need of a well-controlled epidemiological evaluation.

The Smoking Hazard

Epidemiological data indicate that smoking while driving constitutes a serious safety hazard. It is not clear whether the hazard is due to nicotine, due to some psychological characteristic of the smoking driver, or due to poor car control when smoking while driving. Confirmatory studies are desirable, but in the meantime, we should go ahead and warn the smoking public.

Use of Drugs to Improve Performance

Therapeutic drugs can have beneficial as well as harmful effects on traffic safety. Presently, the emphasis is on not driving after drug use to eliminate the possibility of negative side effects. Drug companies use warning labels for a great variety of drugs, hoping that this will absolve them of any responsibility. The law prohibits driving while under the influence of drugs that inhibit driving performance, but these laws are not and perhaps cannot be enforced.

It is suggested to use the beneficial effects of therapeutic drugs to improve accident survival rate and driving performance in medically impaired drivers. This may be done by means of drug selection, by combination of drugs, or by controlled drug delivery. A person with severe hay fever may not be a safe driver unless the clinical condition is controlled by drugs.

BIBLIOGRAPHY

1. Alcohol Safety Action Project, Progress Report *1:*36, Feb. 1979.
2. Babst, D. V., Newman, S., Gorden, N., and Warner, A.: Driving Records of Methadone Maintenance Patients in New York State. *J Drug,* Issue *4:*285, 1973.
3. Baker, S. P. and Spitz, W. U.: Age Effects and Autopsy Evidence of Disease in Fatally Injured Drivers. *JAMA, 214(9):*1079, 1970.
4. Benjamin, F. B.: The Effect of Marihuana on Driving Performance. In *Current Research in Marihuana.* New York, Acad Pr, 1972.
5. Benjamin, F. B.: The Rehabilitated Drug Addict and Traffic Safety. Commission on Human Rights Hearing on the Employment Problems of the Rehabilitated Addict. New York, Jan. 9, 1973.
6. Benjamin, F. B.: A Review of the Safety Hazard Due to Poor Health, Drugs, and Their Interaction. *Human Factors, 19(2):*127, 1977.
7. Benjamin, F. B., Towsend, J. C., Vinograd, S. P., and Bollerud, J.: Integrated Scoring of Tilt Table Response. *Aerospace Med, 39(2):*158, Feb. 1968.
8. Bewley, T. H.: Drugs and Driving. *The Criminologist, 4(12):*7, 1969.
9. Borkenstein, R. F., Crowther, R. F., Shumate, R. P., Ziel, W. B., and Zylman, R.: *The Role of the Drinking Driver in Traffic Accidents.* Bloomington, Indiana University, Mar. 1964.
10. Buttiglieri, M. W., Gruenette, M., and Thompson, M.: Driving Records of Medical and Surgical Patients. *Perceptual and Motor Skills, 29:*427, 1969.
11. California State Highway Patrol: *The Role of Alcohol, Drugs, and Organic Factors in Fatal Single Vehicle Accidents.* Sacramento, June 1967.
12. Cantor, P. D.: *Traumatic Medicine and Surgery.* Woburn, MA, Butterworths, 1959.
13. Clayton, A. B.: The Effects of Psychotropic Drugs Upon Driving-Related Skills. *Human Factors, 18(3):*241, 1976.

97

14. Damkolt, D. K., Toussie, S. R., Akley, N. R., Geller, H. A., and Whitmore, D. G.: *On the Road Driving Behavior and Breath Alcohol Concentration.* DOT-HS-802-264, 1977.
15. Dunlap and Associates: *Drug Abuse and Driving Performance.* DOT-HS-800-754, Oct. 1972.
16. Eelkema, R. C., Bosseau, J., Koshnick, R., and McGee. C. A.: A Statistical Study on the Relationship Between Mental Illness and Traffic Accidents. *Am J Public Health, 60(3):*459, 1970.
17. Essex Corp.: *Comparison of Alcohol Involvement in Exposed and Injured Drivers.* DOT-HS-400954, 1975.
18. Filkins, L. D.: *Alcohol Abuse and Traffic Safety.* FH-11-6555, June 1970.
19. Haddon, W., Valieu, P., McCarroll, J. R. and Umberger, C. J.: A Controlled Investigation of the Characteristics of Adult Pedestrians Fatally Injured by Motor Vehicles in Manhattan. *Chronic Dis, 14:*655, 1961.
20. Holcomb, R. L.: Alcohol in Relation to Traffic Accidents, *JAMA, 3:*1076, 1938.
21. Hollister, L. E.: Psychotherapeutic Drugs and Driving. *Ann Intern Med, 80(3):*413, 1974.
22. Huntley, M. S.: *Alcohol Influences Upon Closed Course Driving Performance.* DOT-HS-801-096, 1974.
23. Hurst, P. M.: *Epidemiological Aspects of Alcohol and Driver Crashes.* DOT-HS-801-096, 1974.
24. Indiana University, Institute for Research in Public Safety: *The Possible Influences of Licit and Illicit Drugs on Driving Behavior.* DOT-HS-800-613, Dec. 1971.
25. Indiana University, Institute for Research in Public Safety: *Tri-Level Study of the Causes of Traffic Accidents.* DOT-HS-804-3-535-73, TAC, May 1979.
26. Indiana University, Institute for Research in Public Safety: *An Overview of the Drug Driving Problem.* DOT-HS-4-00994, Apr. 1975.
27. Interdepartment Committee on Road Safety (France): Senior Citizen and Road Safety (Translation: W. Appich). Paris, May 10, 1977.
28. Kielholtz, P.: Arzneimittel und Verkehrssicherheit. *Z Allg Medizin, 31(27):*787, 1974.
29. Kilbrick, E. and Smart, R. G.: Psychotropic Drugs and Driving Risk. *J Safety Res, 2(2):*73, 1970.
30. Klein, R. H. and Jex, H. R.: Effects of Alcohol on Critical Tracking Task. *J Stud Alcohol, 36(1):*11, 1975.
31. Klonoff, H.: Marijuana and Driving in Real-Life Situations. *Science, 186(4161):*317, 1974.

32. Legg, N. J., Malpas, A., and Scott, D. F.: Effect of Tranquilizer and Hypnotics on Driving. *Br Med J, 1:*417, 1973.
33. Lucas, G. W. H., Kalow, W., McColl, J. D., Griffith, B. A., and Smith, H. W.: *Quantitative Studies on the Relationship Between Alcohol Levels and Motor Vehicle Accidents.* Proceedings 2d Int. Conf. on Alcohol, Drugs, and Traffic Safety, p. 139, Toronto, 1955.
34. Mannheimer, D. I., Mellinger, G. D., and Balter, M. B.: Psychotherapeutic Drugs. *Calif Med, 109:*445, 1968.
35. McCarroll, R. J. and Haddon, W.: A Controlled Study of Fatal Automobile Accidents in New York City. *J Chronic Dis, 15:*811, 1962.
36. Midwest Research Institute: *The Incidence of Drugs in Fatally Injured Drivers.* DOT-HS-119-1-627, Feb. 1974.
37. Midwest Research Institute: *Drug Use Among Drivers.* DOT-HS-119-2-440, Feb. 1975.
38. Midwest Research Institute: *A Comparison of Drug Use In Driver Fatalities and Similarly Exposed Drivers.* DOT-HS-4-00941, Mar. 1977.
39. Moskowita, H.: Psychological Tests and Drugs. *Pharmakopsychiatrie und Neuropharmakologie, 6(2):*114, Mar. 1973.
40. Moskowitz, H., Hulbert, S., and McGlothlin, W. H.: Marihuana, Effects on Simulated Driving Performance. *Accident Analysis & Prevention, 8:*21, 1976, cont'd *8:*45, 1976.
41. National Commission on Marihuana and Drug Abuse in the United States. U.S. Government Printing Press. 5266-00003, Mar. 1973.
42. National Drug Center: *Driver Medical Data and Driver Record Data.* Durham, NC, Jan. 1, 1974.
43. National Highway Traffic Safety Administration: *Societal Costs of Motor Vehicle Accidents.* DOT-HS-802-119, Dec. 1976.
44. National Safety Council: *Accident Facts.* Chicago, 1978.
45. Nichols, J. L.: *Drug Use and Highway Safety. A Review of the Literature.* DOT-HS-800-580, July 1971.
46. Oregon State Board of Health: *Automobile Driving and Chronic Disease.* Eugene, OR, Mar. 1967.
47. Parry, H. J.: Use of Psychotropic Drugs by U.S. Adults. *Public Health Rep, 33(10):*799, Oct. 1968.
48. Perrine, M. W.: *Alcohol, Drugs and Driving.* Proceedings 6th Int. Conf. on Alcohol, Drugs and Traffic Safety, p. 167, Toronto, 1975.
49. Peterson, C. G.: *Perspectives in Surgery.* Philadelphia, Lea & Febiger, 1972.
50. Pollack, S.: *Drinking Drivers and Traffic Safety.* FH-7099, July

1973.
51. Prouty, R. W. and O'Neill, B.: *An Evaluation of Some Qualitative Breath Screening Tests for Alcohol.* Washington, D.C., Insurance Inst. for Highway Safety, 1971.
52. Research Triangle Institute: *Collection, Analysis, and Interpretation of Data on Relationship Between Drugs and Driving.* DOT-HS-022-1-023, Feb. 1972.
53. Ross, H. L.: The British Road Safety Act of 1967. *J Leg Studies, 2(1):*1, 1973.
54. Salventy, G.: Marihuana and Human Performance. *Hum Factors, 17(3):*229, 1975.
55. Secretary HEW: *Marihuana and Health.* 6th Annual Rep. to the U.S. Congress, Washington, D.C., DHEW 1976.
56. Smith, H. W.: *The Pharmacology of Alcohol and Alcohol Drug Combinations.* Proceedings 4th Int. Conf. Alcohol, Drugs and Traffic Safety. Bloomington, IL, 1966.
57. South Carolina Commission on Alcohol and Drug Abuse: *Drugs and Driving.* Columbia, SC, 1975.
58. Sterling Smith, R. S.: *A Human Factors Comparison Between Motor Vehicle Operators Responsible for Fatal Accidents and a Control Sample.* DOT-HS-3-595, July 1975.
59. Sugerman, A. A., Reilly, D., and Albahary, R. S.: Social Competence and Essential Reaction Distinction in Alcoholism. *Arch Gen Psychiatry, 12:*552, 1965.
60. Turk, R., McBay, A. J., Hudson, P., and Bullaboy, M. M.: *Involvement of Alcohol, Carbon Monoxide, and Other Drugs in Traffic Fatalities.* Proceedings 6th Int. Congr. Alcohol, Drugs, and Traffic Safety, p. 597, Ontario, 1975.
61. University of Michigan: *Report on Alcohol and Highway Safety.* DOT-HS-5-01217, Sept. 1977.
62. U.S. Government, Department of Commerce: *Social Indicators,* 1973.
63. U.S. Government, Department of Commerce: *Statistical Abstracts of the United States,* 1976.
64. Virginia Highway Research Council: *Accident Rates of Drivers With Chronic Medical Conditions.* Richmond, Virginia Dept. Motor Vehicles, 1975.
65. Voas, R. B.: *Alcohol and Highway Safety Countermeasures.* A Report to the National Highway Safety Bureau Priorities Seminar. June 19, 1969.
66. Waller, J. A.: Chronic Medical Conditions and Traffic Safety. *N Engl J Med, 273(26):*1413, 1965.
67. Waller, J. A.: *Medical Impairment to Driving.* Springfield,

Thomas, 1973.
68. Willette, R. E.: *Drugs and Driving, National Institute on Drug Abuse Research*, Monograph 11. DHEW ADM 77-432, 1977.
69. Wilson, J. L.: *Handbook of Surgery*. Los Altos, CA, Lange, 1969.

GLOSSARY

ASAP   *Alcohol Safety Action Program*: a program, launched in 1968 and supported by Federal funds, in which 35 states tried to decrease alcohol involved traffic accidents.

BAC   *Blood Alcohol Concentration*: expressed in terms of grams per 100 milliliters of blood.

DOT   *U.S. Department of Transportation*

DWI   *Driving While Intoxicated*: means driving with a BAC above the legal limits of 0.1 percent BAC.

H.I.   *Hazard Index*: indicated by the relationship of the incidence in accidents to the incidence in the nonaccident driver.

LAS   *Low Accident Survivability*: under clinical conditions is Increased Surgical Risk.

NHTSA   *National Highway Traffic Safety Administration*: one of the 6 groups forming the DOT.

P.I.   *Performance Impairment*: demonstrated under controlled laboratory conditions.

INDEX

A

Accident Survival, 18-23, 25, 26, 71, 75, 77, 80, 81, 87, 91, 94
Advanced age, 19, 21, 25
Alcohol countermeasures, 10, 12, 94
Alcohol-related accidents, 7, 8, 9
Alcohol Safety Action Program, 38
Amobarbital, 84
Amphetamine, 47, 48, 54, 55, 59, 60
Analytical methods, 53
Antihistamines, 50-52, 72, 73, 76, 88
Anxiety, 74
Arthritis, 75, 82

B

Barbital, 59, 60
Blood alcohol concentration, 12, 13, 20, 27, 28, 30, 31, 34, 36-38, 40, 45, 93, 94
Blood brain barrier, 53
Blood drug concentration, 50, 53, 88
Breath, 51

C

Cardio-vascular disease, 74, 75, 83
Cocaine, 46, 47, 59, 60
Cold, 76
Coronary Artery Disease, 82
Corticosteroids, 75
Critical Tracking Task, 28, 31

D

Daytime accidents, 10-12, 18, 56
Decision making, 21, 27, 29, 31-33

Deliriants, 59, 60
Depression, 61, 74
Diabetes, 23, 72, 75, 82, 83, 85
Diazepam, 48
Disposable breath tester, 36
Divided Attention Test, 28, 31
Driving behavior, 57, 58
Driving performance, 4, 21-24, 28, 29, 31, 44, 61, 71, 75-78, 81, 87
Driving simulator, 29, 31
Drugs of abuse, 4, 71, 77
Drug enforcement, 45
Drug hazard, 8
Drunk Driver Warning System, 37

E

Emergency medical care, 18, 19
Enforcement, 45, 72, 92, 93
Epilepsy, 73, 74, 76, 82, 83, 85
Euphoria, 25, 32
Eyeglasses, 78

F

Fatal accidents, 4, 6-12, 19-21, 25, 31, 68, 70
Fatigue, 21, 35, 41
Five year plan, 6
Frequency of driving, 57

G

Grand Rapids study, 11, 12, 14

H

Hallucinogens, 46, 47, 51, 59, 60

Hazard index, 11, 12, 15-17
Heroin, 46, 47, 54, 59
Hypertension, 23, 72, 82

I

Illicit drugs, 46-48, 57, 58, 65
Impairment limits, 43
Information processing, 21
Injury accidents, 6-10, 31
Instrumented car, 30

J

Judgment, 21, 65

L

Lapse of consciousness, 74, 85
Legal limits, 34, 35, 38, 41, 43, 45, 72, 92-94

M

Marihuana, 13, 29, 46-48, 50, 59-61, 64-66, 68, 77, 95
Medical impairment, 35, 71
Mental illness, 74, 82
Methadone, 54, 58-60
Migraine, 72, 76
Motor performance, 84
Muscular coordination, 21, 64

N

Narcolepsy, 75
Narcotic analgesics, 50-52, 55, 56, 61, 95
Nicotine, 51, 52, 68-70, 95
Nighttime accidents, 10, 12, 18
Nitrazapam, 84
Non-fatal accidents, 19, 21, 56
Nystagmus, 36

O

Over the counter drugs, 46-48, 65

P

Parkinson's disease, 75
Pedestrian fatalities, 3
Perception, 21
Perceptive error, 26
Pentobarbital, 54
Performance impairment, 25, 26, 33, 40, 41, 44, 45, 81, 85, 91, 93, 94
Performance testing, 27, 28, 32, 34, 35, 94
Prescription drugs, 47, 48, 65
Property damage accidents, 7-10, 31
Psychoactive drugs, 27, 45, 77, 84

R

Reckless driving, 25, 26, 81, 83
Recognition error, 27
Response time, 21, 32
Risk taking, 21, 68, 69, 83

S

Salicylates, 51, 52, 75
Sedatives, 11, 27, 37, 41, 50-52
Self tester, 39
Societal costs, 6-9
Speeding, 26, 32, 35
Stimulants, 11, 13, 27, 50-52, 61
Sustained drug delivery, 88

T

Therapeutic drugs, 4, 23, 44, 45, 77, 91, 96
Tranquilizers, 11, 27, 47, 51, 52, 72, 77, 83
Tunnel vision, 26

U

Uniform Vehicle Code, 55